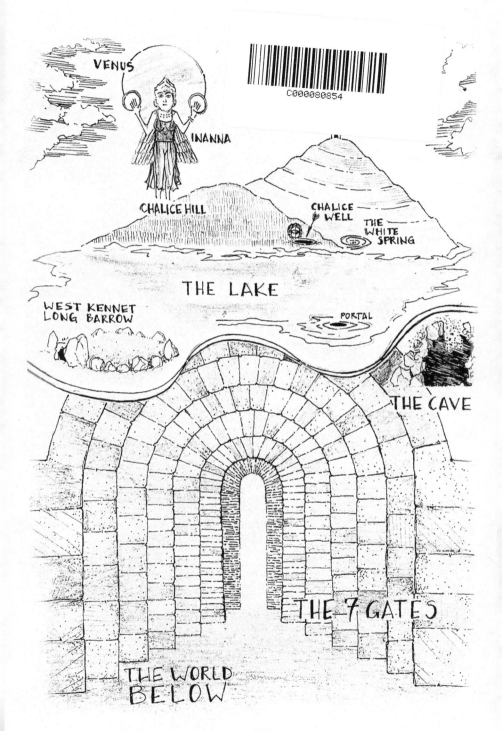

ADVANCE PRAISE

"This magical book of Annah's will inspire you, ground you in mystical tradition, and transport you on a healing journey that will touch your heart and soul. To know Annah's story is nothing short of a gift—an invitation to reflect on your own potential and embrace it with power and grace. The key to physical wellness is spiritual healing, which Annah beautifully exemplifies in this story. Her passion to help others connect to their deepest purpose is the root of why she is thriving today. I hope you share the blessings of this book with everyone you cherish."

~ LISA LEVITT GAINSLEY, lymphatic expert and author of *The Book of Lymph: Self-Care Practices to Enhance Immunity, Health, and Beauty*

"Women sharing their hearts and truth in word form is required and necessary medicine for these times. Thanks for hearing the call, Annah. Thanks for sharing your experience of cancer, of what was revealed, and what was healed, and thanks for gifting us ALL, in the pages of this book, the magic you discovered along the way."

~ LISA LISTER, bestselling author of *Code Red, Witch*, and *Love Your Lady Landscape.*

"Taylor Phinny's journey through breast cancer at thirty-six and the wisdom she amassed is equal parts riveting and instructive. *Lady of the Lake, Rise* is a beautiful treatise on transforming our pain and finding the path to healing."

~ MOLLY BLOOM, author of *Molly's Game*, made into an Oscar-nominated major motion picture

"What determines whether or not one emerges from cancer treatments feeling decidedly whole, purposeful, and joyful? Annah Taylor Phinny's vulnerable story details a spiritual cleansing and rebirth that any cancer journey can bring to those who dive deep within their hearts and souls for true healing."

~ **KRISTI FUNK, MD**, breast cancer surgeon, bestselling author of *Breasts: The Owner's Manual*, and women's health advocate at pinklotus.com

"Annah Taylor Phinny has a transformational story of a mythological journey of awakening and survival, and she tells it uncommonly well. Any initial resistance I may have had to the Priestess of Avalon was swept aside by the quality of her prose."

~ **DAN GERBER**, author of *The End of Michelangelo*

"Annah Taylor Phinny's intuitive knowledge and passion for all things esoteric has touched and enlightened so many. She's one of the most powerful wisdom keepers of our time."

~ **CAMILLA FAYED**, Founder of Farmacy UK and author of *Farmacy Kitchen Cookbook*

"*Lady of the Lake, Rise* is a poetic telling of transformation. The writing is feminine, deep, and true, and so is the journey. I am grateful that Annah Taylor Phinny has so boldly shared her story, and I look forward to hearing more from the Priestess of Avalon."

~ **SHANNYN SOSSAMON**, actress

"As her godfather, I have known Taylor her entire life. From an early age, it was clear that she is an old soul. She was uncommonly loving and kind as a child and always looked for the best in people. Her remarkable spiritual journey is an extension of the path she has been on since birth."

~ **BILL FORD**, Executive Chair of Ford Motor Company

LADY OF THE LAKE, RISE

LADY OF THE LAKE, RISE

A Heroine's Journey through
Cancer to Wholeness

ANNAH TAYLOR PHINNY

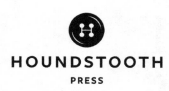

HOUNDSTOOTH
PRESS

LADY OF THE LAKE, RISE

A Heroine's Journey through Cancer to Wholeness

ISBN		
	978-1-5445-3970-6	*Hardcover*
	978-1-5445-3971-3	*Paperback*
	978-1-5445-3972-0	*Ebook*
	978-1-5445-3949-2	*Audiobook*

Lady of the Lake, Rise audio meditations

To access the book's meditations,
read by the author, please visit
https://www.ladyofthelakerise.com/meditations
or use the QR code below.

The recordings include original music
composed by Jerome Zoran.
www.jrokka.com

This book is dedicated to my mother
to all mothers and daughters
and to the healing of our mother lines.

WELCOMING

"To the crossroads I must go
To find a world unseen
Fear and wonder will I know
And be a bridge between."

~ From *To the Crossroads*, by the Reclaiming Tradition,
inspired by a William Butler Yeats poem

Dear Sister, Brother, Friend,

Come with me on a journey
a passage toward remembering what your heart's always known.

As we prepare to embark
take a few moments to breathe, together, deep into our bellies,
releasing audible exhales...*ahhh*.

I stand before you wearing sapphire-colored priestess robes
a crescent moon painted on my brow.

We are in a temple made of stone, the glow of candles flickering
all around us, lush green rolling hills just outside. I light a stick of incense,
and the soothing smell of frankincense fills the air as I begin wafting
its delicate smoke around you with a feather, gently cleansing away the
residue of the outside world, welcoming you into sacred space.

Take off your shoes. Let us walk out into the moonlight,
feeling our bare feet touching the earth. Breathe in the soft, misty air.
Shhhh...quiet...can you hear them?

Voices just under the surface of the wind,
whispering through the mist, calling to you.

In the distance, there is a drumbeat, and enchanted
sounds of women singing.

The waters of the lake are rhythmically lapping on the shore.

The sweet smell of apple blossoms stirs your senses.

Magic is afoot.

CONTENTS

ASCENT

SEVEN GATES OF RECLAMATION

Introduction

THE SPIRAL PATH

NOT A TYPICAL CANCER JOURNEY

"How can I be substantial if I do not cast a shadow?
I must have a dark side also if I am to be whole."

~ Carl Jung

On December 1, 2017, I was diagnosed with breast cancer at age thirty-six. I was sitting on the couch in my mom's living room, my breast bruised and bandaged from the invasive biopsy procedures, riddled with anxiety as I awaited the phone call from the doctor. When the news came, I fell to the floor and screamed. Relentless primal wails flooded through my body from the darkest caverns of the earth, reverberating and echoing through the house like thunder. It was beyond my realm of comprehension at the time that I was crossing a threshold into the most exquisite transformation of my life. I stand before you now, dear reader, to share that I wouldn't trade it for anything.

As I was contemplating how to share my story, I thought about the difference between a hero's journey and a heroine's. The hero's journey is linear, based on outward movement toward a quest, conquering fears, learning a lesson, and coming back to share the wisdom gleaned. The heroine's journey is a spiral, ebbing and flowing, waxing and waning like the moon. As she evolves and grows, she spirals up and down, expanding and opening, awakening to greater levels of self-realization, and simultaneously triggering unconscious wounds that have lain dormant in the shadows. Courageously diving into these dark caverns, the heroine expresses repressed emotions or fears, acknowledges trauma, and shines a light on the darkness, giving it a voice and bringing it into the light. Through this spiraling dance, she awakens to and integrates more and more of the truth of who she is. She reclaims disowned or fragmented pieces of herself, some aspects that have been waiting lifetimes to be seen.

In my experience and understanding, we have lived before, our souls reincarnating in service to our growth, evolution, and remembering our divine nature. The root cause of a wound comes forward in present-time awareness when it is ready to be healed, no matter where or when it originated, be it five years ago, five thousand years ago, or beyond. *For when the heroine heals, she is healing the collective feminine as well.*

We are multidimensional beings who exist eternally, and although we are infinite, we experience limitation within the constructs of time. Time is actually a perception that we have the innate potential to transcend, and in so doing, we may actualize the omnipotence of our divine nature. The heroine's journey is vast, beyond these perceived limitations of time or the human body, and open to embrace all. Her journey accepts all feelings and experiences, all she has been or may be, just as a mother unconditionally loves her child and all that they may or may not become.

Healing is cyclical, layered, and multidimensional. Through the experiences I am about to share, I have come to know this to be true about time, as well. When reading this book, you will notice that the sequence of events is not chronological. I'm sharing from my reality, which shifted from being a scared fifteen-year-old, to an ancient priestess, to a thirty-six-year-old woman with an IV in her arm, all within the same day. My consciousness danced across a spectrum of vibrant, luminous, expansive rainbow hues to cold, frightening, dense shades of gray and black. I saw my life as a blanket, woven with beautiful wool, intricately designed with interweaving colors. Every feeling, memory, and experience overlapped and touched. Following the thread of a feeling, I arrived in a memory, which unraveled into experiences from many different ages, some beyond this lifetime. The threads of these experiences spanned the blanket, and in the interwoven design, I became aware of recurring themes and patterns within my memories and an undeniable organization to the lessons being learned. Everything that arose was here and now, in the present, coming forward to allow for healing to occur deep down at the root. I was not looking back in time, perceiving something outside of me. I was feeling the pain, crying the tears, and expressing the anger in the present moment. The blanket was holding me tightly in a cocoon, reminding me again and again there was nowhere else to look but within. As my eyes adjusted to the dark, I surrendered deeply to the divine path being set before me.

PRIESTESS OF AVALON

I am a Priestess of Avalon in a goddess tradition based in Glastonbury, England. I was beginning the second spiral (year) of a three-spiral (three-year) training when I was diagnosed, which intensely amplified my devotion and dedication to my path. Moving through breast cancer actually felt like part of the curriculum of my training.

A priestess is a woman who lives life in service to the sacred feminine, acting as a vessel for goddess energies to flow into her community. She is a bridge between worlds, helping others open to and experience the realms of the unseen. She offers ceremonies for rites of passage and holy days, practices divination, and offers spiritual support and guidance. She is attuned to the rhythms and cycles of nature, at one with the elements, and receptive to messages from Mother Earth and all her creatures. She interprets life through symbols, archetypes, and metaphors.

A Priestess of Avalon specifically works with the energies, landscape, and mysteries of the ancient Isle of Avalon, which is modern-day Glastonbury, United Kingdom. This sacred landscape is known as the "heart chakra of the earth." There is a potent energy field in present-day Glastonbury/Avalon that bridges the veil of forgetting, the veil that we pass through to navigate everyday human reality. Those of us who feel the irresistible pull to Avalon, the wisdom and memories of our souls—who we were before passing through that veil—are held in this energy field, in the heart of the Goddess. Avalon is known for catalyzing profound transformation in the lives of those who love Her. While the land resonates with a magnificent heart field, one must enter through the shadow of the heart, coming directly into contact with disowned grief, despair, shame, self-pity, anger, rage, resentment, hatred, and disempowerment—all the feelings that most people would prefer to keep hidden. We must first heal our wounds to experience true joy and ecstasy.

The path of the sacred feminine is a path of embodiment. To fully inhabit the landscape of our bodies, we must explore the terrain that has been abandoned or neglected. The more we see, love, and heal within ourselves, the greater pleasure we are able to experience in our bodies and in our lives. The goddess path is about learning to embody our divine nature, bring more of our soul energy into being, and experience life fully through the gift of the senses. *Our bodies are holy vessels for experiencing the sacredness of Her body, which is personified through the earth, and her Spirit, the essence of the divine feminine.*

The Lady of Avalon is a goddess of transformation, healing, death, and rebirth. The ancient Welsh name for the Isle of Avalon was Ynis Witrin, which means Isle of Glass, describing the glassy lake that surrounded the shores. The Lake of Avalon was an enchanted body of water that was reflective like a mirror, revealing what was hidden in the realm of the unseen and triggering what needed to be seen and healed to spiritually transform. The lake was imbued with a divine feminine spirit, known as the Lady of the Lake, who came to me as a personal guide and aspect of my own consciousness during my healing journey. She described herself this way:

> *I am multidimensional. I am personal while also being an archetypal energy. In Avalon, many women have reigned as the Lady of the Lake. All are similar to a reigning queen on a throne. An energy imbues each woman as a whole, and yet each one is a particular emanation that holds significant wisdom and memories relevant to her particular time as the Lady of the Lake.*

Avalon was a sacred island of healing, divination, mysticism, transformation, and magic. The priestesses honored the Goddess in all her forms—her trees, creatures, and the land—as her body. King Arthur's sword, Excalibur, was forged by the priestesses of Avalon, assuring his protection and victory as long as he pledged allegiance with the Goddess of the land, honoring the old ways. There are many legends of Avalon; however, Avalon is not simply a legend whispering echoes of the distant past. Avalon exists purely within the energy field of the ancient landscape that is modern-day Glastonbury. It is a land of shimmering crossroads, with openings in the energetic heart field where one's consciousness may enter the realm of the Holy Isle.

In the priestess tradition I am part of, we pull threads through the misty veils and bring the power of these mysteries into the present. Through walking the land, immersing in the water, and communing with the spirits of the old trees, memories of ancient Avalon are awakened. We honor the sacred landscape as the body of the Lady of Avalon and celebrate the ancient goddesses of the British Isles. My teacher, Kathy Jones, started a goddess temple in Glastonbury. It is the first goddess temple in Europe for more than one thousand years. The foundation of our tradition is the Wheel of Bridannia, the word

"Bridannia" being an ode to the ancient goddess of the British Isles, Brittania, blended with the names of Celtic goddesses Brigid and Ana. This wheel is based on the Celtic wheel of the year, which is comprised of eight seasons. Each season resonates with the energies and qualities of specific goddesses, sacred trees, animals, and more. For those of you interested in discovering more about my priestess tradition, please visit the resources section at the back of the book.

INANNA: MY UNDERWORLD GUIDE

During my cancer experience, when I was lying in bed sick from chemo, nauseated, bald, and bones aching so badly I felt my legs might split in two, an ancient presence relentlessly knocked at my door.

A feminine voice whispered the name, "*Inanna... Inanna... Inanna...*"

She called out to me from the depths of the unknown, "*Sister, follow me...sister, I will show you the way.*"

Her presence grew stronger and her voice louder until I embraced her story of descent into the underworld as a mirror for my experiences. My desire to understand and interpret the messages I was receiving from Inanna initiated my process of writing this book. It was through writing that her voice crystallized, and the profound nature of the lessons I was learning came clearly into focus.

Inanna is an ancient Sumerian goddess who was known as the queen of heaven. Her sister, Ereshkigal, was the queen of the dead who ruled the underworld. In the story of Inanna's descent, she journeys from heaven, to earth, to the underworld to visit her widowed sister. She leaves behind instructions for her faithful servant to come for her if she does not return in three days and three nights. When Inanna arrives in the underworld, she faces seven bolted gates. The gatekeeper commands that she remove one of her royal garments to pass through each gateway. She is stripped of the trappings of the upperworld—all she has identified with—and arrives in the underworld completely naked. She finds Ereshkigal in agony, overwhelmed with grief and rage over the loss of her husband. Ereshkigal kills Inanna and hangs her on a hook. For three days and nights, Inanna's body hangs upside-down in the underworld. When her servant comes looking for her, she encounters Ereshkigal. Inanna's servant sits with Ereshkigal and reflects her feelings back to her; when Ereshkigal moans, the servant moans back, witnessing her in her pain. Thankful for being acknowledged, Ereshkigal allows the servant to retrieve Inanna's body. After being given food and the water of life, Inanna is resurrected. Upon permission to exit the underworld, Inanna reclaims her seven items at each gate, returning to the upperworld where she resumes her reign as the queen of heaven, the same, yet changed.

In this myth, Inanna's experience with her sister is symbolic of the heroine's journey to reclaim her "shadow self." Ereshkigal represents Inanna's shadow, an area of her unconscious comprised of aspects of her psyche that are hidden in the depths of the unknown. Everyone has a shadow and a dark sister or brother inside. What lives here is completely hidden and removed from everyday reality. However, the energies that exist in this domain inform the rest of our behaviors. I imagine the shadow as a dark body of water that lives beneath the landscape of our personalities. Above ground, we have our identities, the things we give value to that make up who we are in the physical world reality—jobs, families, relationships, and social status. The roots of these earthly identifications are fed from the waters of the unconscious shadowy realm. Although we may not know what exists there, we are nevertheless constantly interacting with it.

The shadow is home to disowned aspects of ourselves, parts of us we are ashamed of, experiences we'd rather forget, and tendencies or behaviors we'd rather not look at or are completely unaware of. Some experiences that have been banished to the realm of the shadow have truly been forgotten or blocked out. Our wounds are there, from this life and material we have brought forward to heal from previous incarnations.

The shadow is rich territory because all these places hold our power. It takes energy to keep everything that has been stored in the shadow tightly tucked away. Years, and maybe lifetimes, of protective armor have been built up around the material that is held there. Inanna is stripped of this armor in the form of her possessions, which represent everything she has identified with, so she can face her shadow.

THE SEVEN GATES

I have organized this book into two parts, the descent and the ascent. The descent mirrors the deconstruction of my life as I knew it with Inanna's journey into the underworld, while the gifts this transformation offered me reflect her ascent into the upperworld. Together, we rise like a phoenix from the ashes. The seven gates of the underworld serve as a chariot, a sacred vehicle that carries us together through the ebbs and flows of my story.

These seven gates are significant because they correspond with the seven chakras, the main energy centers of the body. Each chakra is connected with specific organs and bodily functions, as well as different emotions. The experiences Inanna and I have at each of the seven gates of the underworld are connected with these energy centers. Through this journey, we are given the opportunity to accept, honor, and reclaim the aspects of ourselves we had forgotten and left for dead in the underworld. When Inanna and I embrace our darkness, we open to receive the healing potential that is held in the shadow of the underworld.

In *The Hero with a Thousand Faces*, Joseph Campbell interprets the myth of Inanna as the psychological power of a descent into the unconscious, the realization of one's own strength through an episode of seeming powerlessness and the acceptance of one's own negative qualities. I, however, do not refer to these as negative qualities—they are simply a collection of energies that have been judged—by ourselves or others—as bad, wrong, or unworthy. When we compassionately forgive ourselves for these judgments, we untangle the web of shame binding them out of sight and open ourselves to healing. We empower ourselves by taking dominion over these energies and forgiving ourselves, instead of placing them in the hands of another to someday redeem us.

Drs. Ron and Mary Hulnick, my spiritual psychology teachers from the University of Santa Monica (USM), define healing as "the application of loving to the parts inside that hurt." The parts held within the shadow may hurt, but this doesn't mean they are bad, negative, or unworthy of love. In fact, it's the opposite—loving and forgiving them releases them from the dark and restores their purified energy to conscious life. Ultimately when looking through the eyes of the soul, nothing is good or bad; everything is for the experience of learning and remembering our true nature, which is loving.

When I first embarked on a conscious spiritual path in 2006, I didn't like acknowledging the dark. I felt that if I focused my energy there, I would attract or create darkness in my life. Instead, I concentrated on what I perceived as the light, or positive. As I have grown and evolved, I understand there is no light without dark, no day without night, no energy without rest, no growth without a lesson or catalyst. We live in a world of duality. We learn mostly through experiencing discomfort and course correcting. Seeing, acknowledging, and expressing our own darkness is the key to true spiritual growth and transformation. Overly focusing on the positive and not acknowledging the dark is spiritual bypassing—denying emotions or experiences perceived as negative based on the misunderstanding that emotions like anger, sadness, or grief are not spiritual. True spirituality is about authenticity, honesty, and accepting personal responsibility. Robert Masters, a counselor and teacher I have worked with who specializes in shadow work, emphasizes the importance of learning to release "clean anger." He suggests creating space for "conscious rants," where we allow ourselves to let go of these emotions in a supportive environment in which no one is harmed or blamed. It's important to have tools and resources to support inner work within the shadowy realms and to connect with like-hearted people who may serve as sacred witnesses to our journey.

INANNA AND VENUS

Astrologers have connected the myth of Inanna with the planet Venus because Inanna's descent and ascent are reflected in the sky during Venus's synodic cycle (synodic meaning the meeting place of Earth, Venus, and the Sun), which lasts approximately nineteen months. During this cycle, Venus, as a morning star, descends through seven gateways which are reflected in the conjunctions of the waning moon with Venus. She then completely disappears from view, which is the time Inanna spends in the underworld. Venus is then reborn as an evening star, rising on the horizon. Her light grows stronger and more powerful as she ascends back through the seven gateways reflected in the conjunctions of Venus and the waxing moon. Venus is constantly dying to the old and giving birth to higher consciousness. I have always felt a personal connection with Venus, as my astrology chart is ruled entirely—except for my moon in Pisces—by Taurus and Libra, which are both ruled by Venus.

In helping me to understand the influences of Venus, my friend and astrologer, Divine Harmony, explained, "If anyone is a Venusian woman, it would be you, Taylor. You have ten placements in your astrology chart in the Venus-ruled signs of Taurus and Libra, with Venus well placed in your sensual, embodied sign of Taurus. It's fascinating that you have all your Taurus planets in the eighth house, which is naturally the Scorpio-ruled house. Where Taurus is about beauty, value, acquisition, and abundance, Scorpio is about loss and renewal, death and rebirth, shadow work and transformation."

Understanding the map of my birth chart expands my perception of reality because it describes the ways in which planetary energies influence my life. Inanna's presence in my life during such a painful time felt even more potent when I understood the significance of my astrological placements ruled by the planet Venus in the domain of the underworld, initiation, and transformation. My link with Inanna is right there, written in the stars.

JOURNAL ENTRIES

You will notice that journal entries appear at the end of each chapter in this book. Journaling was an anchor point for me throughout my journey and a practice I highly recommend, especially for those moving through trauma or intensity. The act of putting pen to paper is incredibly cathartic, evoking a sense of peace, a connection to the eye of the storm within the swirling emotions of the inner world. I noticed that simply seeing my experiences outside of me, written on paper, not only validated them but also somehow made them less scary. It gave me a sense of control when everything else felt completely uncontrollable.

Included in my journal entries are dreams I had during treatment. Writing down my dreams upon waking each morning allowed for many insights to rise from the waters of my unconscious. The unconscious speaks in symbols and metaphors, and capturing these images opened a doorway through which I was able to more deeply understand the narrative of my soul's journey. Pulling threads up from the dream realm and writing them in my journal built a bridge between the world of my unconscious and waking reality. And to my amazement, as you will see later in the book, the symbols and images I recorded began showing up in my outer life, signs that I interpreted as confirmations from the Divine that I was on the right path.

Because journaling was profoundly supportive for me, I have included journal prompts for you at the end of each chapter, followed by a meditation. This process will assist you in integrating the learning I gleaned through my healing journey into your own life. When working with the meditations, if you find it difficult to visualize the imagery, relax, and simply set the intention to experience what is being shared. Energy flows where intention goes.

HEALERS ALONG THE WAY

There was an extraordinary team of beings who supported me while I was going through treatment, each with their unique approach. This included an oncologist, a breast surgeon, and a reconstructive surgeon. They provided the traditional Western approach to cancer treatment, which was exactly what I needed on the physical level. However, Western medicine did not address the complex layers of mental, emotional, and spiritual recovery, which, for me, is the path to true healing and wellness. The beings that supported this aspect of my journey included a spiritual healer, an ascended spirit guide channeled through a trance medium, a counselor who specializes in meditation and brainwave optimization, an acupuncturist, Mother Nature, my personal spirit guides, and many more. I have included resources to explore some of these alternative pathways to healing, as well as information about my priestess tradition, Inanna and Ereshkigal, the seven chakras, and the Venus astrology reference in the Resources section at the back of the book.

WHY I WROTE THIS BOOK

This book is for anyone who has been diagnosed with any form of illness or has experienced a trauma in their life. It is an ally for souls working through pain, grief, or despair, or for those holding space for loved ones moving through this type of terrain. I know the feeling of yearning for deeper answers and the profound desire to feel connected to a higher level of understanding. I am familiar with the kind of pain that medical doctors do not have a term for, which is psychic, or spiritual, pain. I have felt the wounds of my ancestors, the weight of persecution and suppression from my soul's past, calling out to me, alive in my body, asking to be remembered.

As an initiated priestess with a background in spiritual psychology, I was able to move through my healing journey with a very unique set of skills. My spiritual understanding and orientation to life provided me with tools to glean great insight into the deeper layers of my experiences and ultimately share them in service to your healing. Through the nonlinear, cyclical storytelling of my book, I forge a path for you to glean awareness and insight into your own heroine's journey. This book will open a gateway for you to experience a multidimensional and holistic way of approaching healing, one that will resonate deep in your bones. You will receive a framework through which you may experience your own healing as a path to wholeness.

Anyone who has faced a life-threatening diagnosis is familiar with the feeling of being plunged into a dark abyss, staring out into the unknown with no map or flashlight. If you are in this place now, dear reader, my prayer is that this book will support you in attuning to your own inner compass. May it serve as a guide that awakens your inner Sight, shifting your perspective so that you may see the divine blueprint laid out before you. May it bring light to your journey and open your heart to new possibilities. As you stand at this threshold, I offer a prayer that is spoken in my priestess tradition when one comes upon a crossroad.

I give thanks for the path that brought me here.

I give thanks for the path I am not choosing.

I give thanks for the path ahead, the path that I am choosing.

Blessed be.

Descent

SEVEN
BOLTED
GATES

Chapter One

UNVEILING CEREMONY

FIRST GATE: BEAUTY

"Beauty is life when life unveils her holy face.
But you are life and you are the veil."

~ Kahlil Gibran

Today is the day I'm losing my hair. I'm standing outside the house we've rented in Topanga, California, feeling displaced, yet at home, in the canyon. In my hands, I'm holding an earthen clay bowl, filled with water for the ceremony my spiritual sisters, beloved husband, and I have created to mark the loss of my hair. Into the ceremonial bowl, I've added drops of water from the lands of my ancestors—from the Red and White Springs in Glastonbury, England; from Brigid's Well of Eternal Youth on the highest point of the Isle of Iona, Scotland; and from Brigid's Well in Kildare, Ireland—all ancient holy places that connect me with my spiritual lineage. As I breathe in the crisp California winter air, I walk toward a beautiful pink, green, and blue floral tapestry my sisters have laid on the earth within a clearing of live oaks.

It's been three months to the day since Blue, my beloved horse, died. I miss him so much it hurts like an open wound. There are horses in this neighborhood and I occasionally hear the clicking of their feet on the pavement as they head for the trail or an excited whinny at dinnertime carried across the breeze. This makes me feel desperately alone, an aching hole in my heart. Not a day has passed in the last three months that I haven't cried for Blue.

My friends have placed a circle of sheepskins around the tapestry, with one sheepskin in the center, a place lovingly created for me to sit, as though I'm a goddess. My seat is surrounded with white and pink roses, quartz and rose quartz crystals, all emanating their pure healing frequencies. Greenery lines the outer circle. It's breathtaking. I carefully set the bowl of water down before the seat in the center, which is waiting for me. Still standing, I take my place in the circle with my husband and five dear sisters surrounding me. I feel my body trembling; I'm scared. I reach for my drum, fingers clinging to the mallet in anticipation of what's next. I close my eyes and see the apple trees in Avalon, from which this wooden beater is made. I rub the drum to warm her up; she's made from red deerskin from the Scottish Highlands. My drum and the holy waters are bringing me great comfort. I can feel the power of the Celtic lands supporting me.

My hair is long, thick, flowing, and hangs past my waist. I am used to receiving compliments about its beauty. I've realized over the last several weeks that my hair has unconsciously been part of the way I have defined myself as a woman, in particular a "goddessy," feminine woman. Long hair lends itself to the social construct of a spiritual, earth-loving woman. There are so many associations automatically placed upon women related to their hair. The color and style of a woman's hair can reveal the way she feels inside, her innermost emotions and traits, perhaps even those rooted in her unconscious. A woman's hair reflects how she desires to be seen, and more deeply, the way she carries the energy of her "spiritual frequency," as the crown chakra vibrates at its roots.

In Kundalini yoga, hair is seen as an antenna for receiving prana, or life force energy, and yogis grow their hair as long as possible. Some Native American tribes also viewed their hair as a channel that attuned them to the subtler energies of the natural world, and believed if their hair was cut, this connection would be weakened or lost. In medieval times, a woman's hairstyle reflected her social status. It was appropriate for maidens to wear their hair free and unbound; however, married women were required to tie their hair back or cover their head with a shawl. Tales of enchantresses often depict them with long, flowing hair, associating them with wild, untamed, and magical power. Energetically, I experience my hair as a form of security blanket. It provides a layer of protection above my crown, a buffer between my spiritual energy center and the outside world.

OUTER HEALING: MEDICAL

When I was receiving my diagnosis, I cried to my doctor, explaining to her that I didn't want to do chemo. She said reassuringly, "We'll just put that beautiful hair in a cold cap." Oh, I was so relieved!

Cold caps are a method of freezing the roots of your hair while receiving a chemo infusion to try to prevent hair loss. This involves sitting with a freezing head for about five hours. I was disappointed to learn the statistics; most women who underwent a cold cap saved about 50 percent of their hair. Still, I tried it, clinging to the hope that it would work well for me, and I would keep more than 50 percent of my hair. Most importantly, I felt the preservation of my physical appearance would allow me to keep my experience private. If I had hair, no one had to know what I was going through. It's funny the things I imagined I would be doing while enduring cancer treatment. The first thing I thought of was going to a yoga class, or out for breakfast with friends, and of course, I never pictured myself bald.

The cold cap was the closest thing to torture I've experienced in this lifetime. It was painfully tight with a strap that pulled forcefully around my chin, clenching my jaw so harshly I could barely open my lips enough to sip through a straw. My head was pounding and heavy from the weight of the cap as tubes connected to the machine sent freezing water over my skull. I could hear and feel a loud swishing as the tubes pulled my head awkwardly down to the side. I sat in this unnatural position, enduring severe discomfort, for about five hours. When it was finally removed, my head was covered in icicles and a thick indent on my forehead reminded me of the tightness of the cap for the next twenty-four hours. I realized in the days and weeks that followed that I was dreading having to go back and sit with that cap on my head, possibly recoiling from the thought of the bone-chilling cap even more than getting chemo!

WISDOM

I thought about the wisdom shared by one of my spiritual teachers, Chung Fu, an ascended spirit guide, channeled through a trance medium in Glastonbury named Sally Pullinger. Chung Fu's perspective is vast and instantly transformative, as he is communicating from "beyond the veil." His wisdom transcends the mind or the human experience, which enables direct connection with the soul. The day after I was diagnosed, he told me that cancer is a dis-ease of suppression and that for my healing, it was imperative to unleash previously suppressed parts of me, to let it all out. If I could imagine a visual that epitomized this feeling of suppression, especially suppression that shut me down spiritually, it was a tight, weighted, painful cap that froze my head.

Just before my second round of chemo, I sat with my dear friend Val in her living room, together feeling into the possibility of discontinuing the use of the caps. Standing across from each other with our eyes closed, she spoke aloud, "Receive the way it feels for Taylor to continue using the cold caps."

I shuddered as my body constricted. I felt tight, withdrawn, and powerfully shut down. Looking at Val's posture, leaning back as if she had been punched in the stomach, I knew she felt the same. It took a moment to shake this off. When we felt clear again, she said, "Receive the way it feels for Taylor to stop using the caps."

An explosion of light burst from my forehead and crown, and I was filled with a surge of divine energy. I felt strong, confident, and empowered. I looked up at Val and her energy field seemed larger than life, radiant with excitement and possibility. It was clear to me in that moment that to really lean into this experience I was facing, to dive into the depths of the healing opportunity that was being presented to me, I needed to own this transformation. If I am desperately clinging to this limited idea of who I think I am, "a goddess-loving woman with long flowing hair," how will I grow and expand and become who I am meant to be?

In one of our first meetings, my oncologist told me that when diagnosed with cancer, most people cry and process a little bit in the beginning, but then power up for treatment, focused on the goal of completing it and returning to their lives. These people have the most difficult time after treatment because they're not only processing all they've just been through, but they've realized they can't go back to who they were before. *There's no going back.* Whether they consciously relate to it as never going back or not, they will have been profoundly changed by the experience and *everything* will be different. A deep grieving happens in this stage as well as a grappling with how to move on.

If cancer is here to transform my life, there is no going back to the woman with long, flowing hair, anyway. *Who will I be on the other side?* In the face of losing a part of my beauty, I'm going to create a beautiful ceremony to honor this transition.

INNER HEALING

When the day comes, I am not alone with clippers crying in the bathroom. Rather, I am held by my husband and sisters, among the beautiful oak trees, my Avalonian lineage, and the spirit of the canyon. Trembling, I begin to hit the beater in my hand against my drum, and I hear myself asking my loved ones to turn to face the northeast. The northeast is the direction of the maiden Brigid.

Brigid, maiden goddess of healing, be with me today as I cross this threshold. Light your flame of inspiration within my heart as I walk through this journey of transformation. Cradle my inner child, her innocence and purity, in your arms.

Mother of fire, Artha, goddess of protection and transmutation, bring me your courage, strength, and ferocity. Burn away old conditioning and limiting beliefs, anything that no longer serves me in this journey. Surround me with the protective flame of Avalon.

Rhiannon, goddess of love and sensuality, help me feel love for myself in every cell of my body. Awaken my sovereignty as a priestess. May the sweet nectar of your unconditional love fill my breasts and heart.

Mother of water, Domnu, goddess of compassion and intuition, cleanse my mind, body, and spirit. Purify my emotions; may they flow with grace and gentleness so that I may be receptive to the wisdom within.

Mother goddess, Ker, great mother of nurturing, please hold me in your tender, loving embrace. Bless my breasts with your life-giving nourishment. Bring your motherly love to any parts of me that have been unmothered. I pray for healing for my mother line.

Mother of earth, Banbha, goddess of stability and manifestation, ground and support me. I call on the power of your standing stones, the dragon lines in the earth of Avalon, and the spirit of this canyon. Please support me in actualizing total and complete healing.

Keridwen, dark goddess of transitions and letting go, you are the keeper of the cauldron of transformation, the guardian between worlds. I feel myself falling into the underworld, into the depths of the unknown. Please be with me, hold me in your cauldron. May I release all that I am meant to, from all levels of consciousness, to heal completely. May I let go with grace and courage. May I surrender to the transformation occurring. I call on my ancestors who support me, my ancestors of blood and spirit.

Mother of air, Danu, goddess of peace, blow your winds of change around me, cleanse and clear away any misunderstanding, negativity, or stagnation from my mind and heart. Bring me your insight; may I see and understand all that is unfolding from a higher perspective.

Beloved Lady of Avalon, goddess of death, rebirth, and transformation, wrap me in your rainbow light. May I remember the mysteries, magic, and power of my ancient priestess self. May I awaken fully to the wisdom that is available to me during this time of initiation. I know you are guiding me, Lady. I thank you, and I love you. Blessed be.

I kneel down and place my hands upon the earth, offering the energy moving through me to the land with gratitude. My husband, sisters, and I take our seats and my friend Harmony steps forward, anointing me with sacred oils of frankincense, myrrh, and spikenard. She speaks blessings into my seven chakras and says, "I love you, and I will walk through the fire with you."

My friend and spiritual counselor, Alisha, blesses my crown with holy water, speaking powerful words of prayer. Val steps forward, holding a seashell filled with blue paint. The cool brush in her hand creates patterns on my face, stirring a deep sense of familiarity within me. A crescent moon at my brow, a spiral on my chin, and lines around my eyes light up my face with otherworldly power. Staring at me with fire in her eyes, Val declares me a warrior priestess. A power washes over me, the power of acceptance. *I have cancer.* And I know that I'm ready for this initiation.

My sisters, Jenny and Keri, whisper blessings of strength, courage, and unconditional love into my ears. I can feel the grounded, comforting presence of my husband, Ryan, sitting behind me.

"Alright, it's time for Excalibur," he says.

We had jokingly named the clippers Excalibur, and I welcome the temporary comic relief. I know Ryan is nervous, and I can feel his hands trembling at the nape of my neck. The buzzing of the clippers is all-encompassing, deafening for a moment. I take a deep breath and clench the beater of my drum. *What do I do?* I haven't thought about what to do during this part of the ceremony. My body is shaking as I feel the cold clippers at the top of my forehead, buzzing backward over my scalp. A lock of hair falls onto my arm, and I instinctively let out a cry. I've always hated getting my hair cut. Even when my hair was down to my waist, I'd get anxious about trimming off an inch. I begin playing my drum, swaying, and crying. I feel Keri's hands holding my head steady as my body rocks.

Noises are coming out of me, songs of flowing soul language, tones of an unknown tongue coming up from somewhere deep inside my grieving soul. As I feel more of my hair fall to the ground, the songs turn into cries, and then screams. I feel a deep power within as screams, wails, and laughs rhythmically flow through me. There is a palpable energy field swirling around us; we have all entered this sacred space together. As I am expressing myself, my friends are mirroring me, singing and humming as I sing, screaming with me, shedding tears as I am crying. We are tapping into something much bigger, something archetypal, a collective experience of women's anguish, pain, release, and also celebration. As I cry, I feel the sobs of women who haven't been "witnessed" or held in their pain. As I rejoice, I feel the honoring of women who have not been seen or acknowledged in their triumphs. I feel Ereshkigal in the underworld, and the healing she experiences when her moans of agony are echoed back to her.

The buzzing stops. My friends look at me with awe and wonder.

"How is it possible for you to be even more beautiful?" Val asks.

I turn to face Ryan, tears streaming down my face. I have never felt more vulnerable, more exposed. He says, "Your hair was beautiful, my love, but it hid the enormousness of your beauty. Now I can really see you. You look gorgeous."

Tears, fully released, continue to flow down my face. My friends shower me with compliments. Alisha lifts the bowl of sacred waters and washes my newborn head. *If I can do this, I can do absolutely anything.*

My hair looks strange to me, laying in a blonde heap on the earth like the fur of an otherworldly animal that has just passed—this hair that has brought me so much suffering and has represented so much. As I stare at my lost tresses, piled lifeless at my feet, I feel stronger and more powerful than ever before. I collect my hair into a bag, unsure of what I'll do with it. Ryan wraps me in a blanket and leads me inside, my sisters cleaning up the ceremonial site. I place my hair on my altar, alongside Blue's tail, for now.

INANNA

Gate 1: Removal of Her Crown: Beauty

As Inanna enters the underworld and knocks at the outer gates, she's greeted by the chief gatekeeper. Having left her seven temples on Earth, adorned in her royal garments, she's going to visit her recently widowed sister, Ereshkigal. When the gatekeeper gives Ereshkigal the message that Inanna has arrived, she's furious and commands that Inanna be stripped of her royal garments at each gate.

"Let the holy priestess of heaven enter bowed low," she says.

There are seven gateways leading into the underworld, mirroring the seven temples on Earth above. At the first gate, the gatekeeper commands Inanna relinquish her crown, stripping her of her identity as the queen of heaven. The physical crown rested in the space of her crown chakra, the energy center at the top of the head. The crown chakra is a place of connection with universal energy and higher consciousness. For Inanna, her crown served as a link to her sense of self as a goddess and queen. Removing the adornment of the crown leaves her feeling stark, exposed, isolated, uncomfortable, no longer safely protected by what it represented—her royal status. As I walk through the first gate of the underworld, I must surrender my identity as a beautiful woman: the long, flowing hair from my crown and all that represented to me. I am frightened of being ugly, unattractive, unfeminine, and isolated from the woman I have been. My husband loved my long blonde hair.

Dream Journal Entry, One Week before Losing Hair

I'm drinking a potion that makes my hair disintegrate into dust. Like Gwynevere (when the monks of Glastonbury Abbey opened her tomb, her perfectly intact golden hair turned to dust). I'm thrilled when this happens. I'm walking in the woods and am given this potion in a small clay jar to drink. The potion is sparkling and effervescent yet like clay or mud at the same time.

Dream Journal Entry

Dreamed about having dark energy on my hair and needing to get rid of it. I was with a woman who was explaining this to me; she cut my braid off with a sword. My hair had a speck of blood on it. Later, this woman was preparing a bath of black water for me to cleanse in.

JOURNAL PROMPT

What status do you identify with in your life? How might you be "wearing this" status energetically as a way of identifying who you are to the outside world? What validation do you receive?

MEDITATION

Sit comfortably with your spine straight, or lie down, where you will not be disturbed.

Close your eyes, and begin taking in deep diaphragmatic breaths, in through the nose, filling and expanding the belly, and out through the mouth with an audible exhale...ahhh. Repeat three times.

When you feel centered, focus your awareness at your crown, the energy center just above the top of your head. This center connects you with your higher Self. Breathe here for a few moments with the intention of sensing the subtle vibration of energy and visualizing the color violet.

Ask yourself: "What have I identified with in my life that disconnects me from my true essence?"

Allow yourself to receive whatever impressions, symbols, memories, feelings, or insights that pop into your awareness. If this sense of identification could be encapsulated in a symbol, what would that symbol be?

Once you have the symbol in your mind's eye, visualize the goddess Inanna standing before you. She has a regal presence: tall with long, dark hair and deep brown eyes. Dressed in her royal robe, she is carrying her scepter (or staff) and adorned in her gold bracelet, a copper breastplate, a lovely string of beads, and a lapis necklace. She is no longer wearing her crown.

Bringing your symbol once more into your mind's eye, see yourself handing it over to Inanna with the intention of releasing any false sense of identification that keeps you separate from your truest sense of Self. Inanna carries this symbol with her across the threshold of the first gate of the underworld.

As you witness her walking away, feel the release of what this has represented in your life. How does it feel to let go? Who are you without this? Allow yourself to be present with any thoughts or feelings that arise.

When you are ready, return to your breath, repeating the three deep diaphragmatic breaths we began with.

Slowly open your eyes and take a moment to journal any insights that came forward.

Blessed be.

Chapter Two

THE DESCENT

SECOND GATE: MY MAGICAL NATURE

*"Edges, it seems, breed edges; and journeys, like edges,
are fractal. There is never just one."*

~ Sharon Blackie

I am always amazed at the power of the unconscious, at our ability to know things before we actually know them consciously. For example, a few months before my grandfather was killed in a car accident, he began recalling his childhood in incredible detail—the bike he rode around the neighborhood at age seven and favorite meals his mother prepared. I have heard similar stories of elders who became more sentimental in the months approaching their death, telling previously unheard stories of their lives to loved ones. I was particularly struck by this phenomenon manifesting in my grandfather because, on a physical level, his death was perceived as a sudden accident. His soul, however, knew. Our souls always know.

In our modern Western culture, the concept of death is avoided at all costs, yet our ancestors understood it to be a natural and integral part of the cycle of life. Death was honored as a sacred transition.

Birth and death were seen as gateways into the realm of Spirit. Celts believed that our souls traveled to and from the Otherworld, a place of renewal and healing, within the larger journey of the soul, which is a continuous circle. Death was not seen as an ending but rather as a necessary transition to become something else. Within the Celtic wheel of the year, Samhain (pronounced Saw-ain), is simultaneously the ending and beginning of the year. This exemplifies the age-old understanding that one does not exist without the other. Samhain was seen as a time to release things from our lives that were no longer needed, and to set intentions for the year ahead. As the fall leaves descended from the trees and returned to the earth for regeneration, they carried the energy of resolutions made at Samhain. After a period of gestation in the darkness of winter, they were reborn with the new light and life of spring.

Within the cycles of our lives, we experience death as a rite of passage, as an ending phase of life, as a release of one way of being to become something else or to enter our next phase of evolution. We shift through many endings in our lives: completing school, ending relationships, moving our place of residence, changing jobs, the ending of one year and the welcoming of the next each year on a birthday. When a new cycle begins, some part of us dies to make room for the changes it brings. These parts of us that are released go through a process of transformation to be reborn.

Looking back at the months before I was diagnosed with breast cancer, I am astonished at the level of soul-knowing that was pouring forth. I was completing the first year of my three-year Priestess of Avalon training in Glastonbury on the autumnal equinox.

SISTER OF AVALON

I am standing barefoot on the cold earth of Avalon. The moon is a perfect silver waxing crescent, my favorite kind of moon. As the fire rages in the center of our circle, my ears delight in the sounds of several owls in the trees above, hooting in a chorus around me. There is a priestess embodying the Goddess, serving as a conduit to bring forward Her divine energy so that initiates may communicate directly with Her. As I kneel before this cloaked and masked priestess, I speak my vows of dedication:

I ask to clearly receive your guidance as I step forward on this path.

I ask for your support in remembering Avalon and who I am.

I offer my loving devotion as your clear channel.

May you bless and strengthen my relationship with my beloved, and all family and friends, so that through their reflection I may grow into the woman I am meant to be.

I will serve your highest good and the highest good of all concerned.

I dedicate myself as a Sister of Avalon.

Blessed be.

I am adorned in a blue-and-gold gown that I first saw in a vision while standing in a stone circle overlooking a loch (Scottish for "lake") in the Scottish Highlands, just three months before. In this vision, a feminine water spirit appeared, emerging from the loch and walking toward me, dripping with water and mud. As she moved closer, she became the Lady of the Lake, adorned in a sapphire-blue gown with a golden crescent moon crown above her head. Wielding the sword in her hand, she began removing layers of net from my etheric body. I felt as though I had been caught in a fisherman's net out at sea without knowing it. This etheric web of ropes and netting fell in heaps around my feet. She instructed me to wear a blue-and-gold dress to my dedication ceremony.

Weeks later, as I sat at my computer searching for this dress, I stumbled upon a medieval costume designer. A fairy godmother's wand may have emerged from the screen as my finger clicked on an image because what happened next was truly magical. There it was: a beautiful blue-and-gold dress actually named "the Lady of the Lake."

As I stand in this gown during my ceremony, I feel the power of something ancient activating within me with such force I shudder slightly with fear. Raising my arms high into the night sky, I close my eyes and feel the words clearly written on my heart: *I'm ready.* As the other initiates and I walk silently in the night from the site of the ceremony, one of them whispers to me, "I looked up at you standing by the fire tonight and thought, 'My God, I am looking at the Lady of the Lake.'" I went to sleep that night feeling expansive and joyful, knowing that my life had been changed.

I awake the next morning with overwhelming feelings of dread and anxiety. I've started bleeding, which I am expecting, and it's normal for my moon time to be accompanied by physical pain and heaviness. This emotional experience feels different, however. Fears are creeping up from unknown depths and filling my mind with all kinds of horrors. The most gripping, unshakable fear is telling me that I have a dis-ease. As if placed on a platter at the forefront of my awareness, a memory is crystallizing. I hear the words spoken by a naturopath in Encinitas. "Your white blood cell count is elevated," she said. "Have you been sick recently?" I answered no. "Your body is probably fighting off an infection," she responded. "I wouldn't worry about it. You're so healthy."

I began to panic at the sudden recall of a conversation that had previously gone in one ear and out the other. *What does a high white blood cell count mean?* I began googling hepatitis C, obsessively thinking about a small tattoo I'd gotten on my wrist in my early twenties. *I didn't like the feel of that place*, I thought. *Why did I go there?*

Overwhelmed by anxiety, unfamiliar territory, and a door I didn't want to open, I close the computer and breathe deeply. I soothe myself by concluding that I'd experienced such significant expansion in the ceremony that previously unseen and well-hidden shadows were being revealed.

RELEASING WEIGHT

I remember one of my teachers, Dr. Ron Hulnick, describing the layers of a person's consciousness. He drew a graph of the unconscious, physical, emotional, mental, and spiritual levels, showing all the material being evenly dispersed between them. When one level shifts dramatically, such as when a person releases weight physically, all the other layers have to reorganize themselves and the equal amount of spiritual, mental, emotional, and unconscious material will come forward to be released as well. He shared that this is why people often put weight back on, because they haven't done the inner work along with the outer. *This is all good!* I thought. I am expanding spiritually. Anything not in alignment with this spiritual elevation and expansion needs to come up and out. This fear is masking a sense of unworthiness, a feeling that there must be something wrong with me, that I'm not good enough. These feelings are manifesting in the form of this idea of dis-ease. *Okay, this makes sense to me.*

I write in my journal, go for a walk, even try curling up in bed and watching an episode of *Outlander*. But I can't shake this feeling of dread. It feels different than anything that has come up before. As much as I try to work with the feelings and cultivate a space of self-healing, I am experiencing total anxiety, panic, and a sense of impending doom. Not what I expected after the bliss of my dedication ceremony!

KATHY JONES, FOUNDER OF THE GODDESS TEMPLE

The next day, I walk to the Goddess House for a healing session with Kathy Jones, the "creatrix" of the priestess program and Founder of the Glastonbury Goddess Temple. When I made the appointment, I'd been excited to connect with her, as she would one day be my teacher. As I sit before her now, I feel embarrassed that I cannot stop crying.

"I think I'm having old shame come up as I'm being seen and received in such a pure way by this community," I share. "All of my insecurities are coming up. I used to do drugs and abuse my body in my early twenties, and I have a lot of shame around that."

Why am I telling her this in our first conversation? She asks me to put my hands on the place in my body where I feel this and to give the feeling a voice.

"I feel like I'm waiting for the other shoe to drop," I say. "That something bad is about to happen."

Louise Hay uses that phrase "waiting for the other shoe to drop" in her book *You Can Heal Your Life* as she describes the thought pattern underlying the physical experience of shingles. When I had shingles and read Louise Hay's words, I hadn't connected with them. But I did now.

At the end of our session, Kathy tells me she felt I had a lot of repressed anger. "You're a very nice person, and nice people often have a lot of anger," she says.

This was a reflection I'd never heard before. I'd been doing deep inner work for ten years at this point, including completing a masters' program in spiritual psychology at USM with an emphasis in consciousness, health, and healing. Essentially, this was three years immersed in transformational therapy. Friends and I half-jokingly referred to it as "crying school" because of the amount of processing and experiential work it involved. My boyfriend at the time used to feel uncomfortable at how nonchalantly I would cry or express my emotions in public. For the majority of these last ten years, I had also apprenticed with a powerful and fierce healer named Nicholas, an exorcist who constantly challenged me, and I had received countless trainings in yoga, ritual work, and healing modalities.

As I sit before Kathy, speaking of my repressed anger, however, I feel like a novice. I'm swimming in unfamiliar dark waters, my feet are searching for the sand below, yet the water only gets colder, and the bottom is out of reach. I breathe deeply and know Kathy is on to something.

. . .

During the next month of October, at home in California, the feelings of dread and dis-ease stay with me. The wheel of the year is turning toward Samhain, the time of the year ruled by the dark goddess, the crone, and the wise woman archetype. It's a time to connect with the wisdom of our ancestors and beloved dead. It's a time of shedding and letting go, of transformation, death, and rebirth. Samhain, celebrated on October 31 and November 1, is the origin of Halloween. I'm preparing to offer a public ceremony in honor of Samhain before I travel to Avalon to begin the second spiral of my training.

Only a few brave souls—mostly friends—show up to support me for my Samhain ceremony. I find this lack of participation to be an interesting and clarifying reflection of our collective fears versus what feels safe. The Beltane ceremony I'd offered the previous May in honor of the goddess as lover, focusing on sensuality, love, and pleasure, had generated lots of interest and strong attendance. But for Samhain, we celebrate the dark goddess, who is the literal opposite of the goddess as lover and sits on the other side of the wheel. The dark goddess reigns in the season of the year when things are shedding as opposed to blossoming. She is the unknown.

Shadow figures dance on the walls of the candlelit room as I invoke the dark goddess, Keridwen. Beating my drum, I ask that she help me release all that no longer serve my highest expression into Her cauldron of transformation. We sang to Her, *Keridwen, Keridwen, dark goddess, take us in, Keridwen, Keridwen, let us be reborn.* I guide everyone on a vision journey to meet Keridwen in Her medicine cave. Sitting before Her cauldron, she stirs the bubbling liquid, occasionally dropping in different herbs, preparing the healing medicine each woman needs. She looks up, her ancient eyes brimming with wisdom, and asks, "Are you ready to drink of my brew?"

BLUE'S PASSING

Three days later, on October 24, my beloved horse and soul companion, Blue, fell ill with colic during a heat wave. Nine years earlier, when I'd rescued his majestic soul from a string of abandonments and negligent owners who had left him injured and in pain, I'd felt a connection so powerful that I knew we were actually *reuniting* from a past life.

He was very stiff and could barely walk when I rescued him; people around the neighborhood in Topanga referred to him as crippled. I saw only the radiance of his spirit and the strength and resilience of his body. I'd found him as I was driving up to a healing horse ranch to inquire about an apprenticeship. I was in my second year of USM and wanted to learn equine therapy. I had grown up with horses; we had eight of them at my childhood home, one of whom had three foals before I was ten. One of my favorite childhood memories is my mom waking me up in the middle of a hot, balmy Michigan summer night with excitement, saying, "Hannah had her baby!" I ran down to the barn in my pajamas to see her beautiful foal awkwardly taking her first steps.

I rode English and began show jumping at the tender age of seven. From ages sixteen to twenty-seven, I didn't have contact with horses, and by the time I was at USM, I missed them desperately. When I drove past Blue for the first time, I pulled off the road to pet him and my heart burst with loving recognition. He was the most beautiful horse I had ever seen. A palomino, he had a perfect honey-colored coat, a white mane and tail, and a white star on his forehead. I decided the star was where his horn used to be. Blue became my gateway to my magical self, to the young girl within who trusted her perception of the spirit world.

My times with Blue were the most sacred moments of my days. Being out on the land with him, among the rocky landscape and fields of sagebrush, I'd sing and chant goddess songs, allowing my most private inner self to emerge. *The earth, the air, the fire, the water, return, return, return, return*. We went on full-moon rides—just the two of us—and once, on a cloudy night, we were entrenched in such sheer darkness that I couldn't even see the trail before me. I closed my eyes and trusted Blue would safely bring me home, and he did. Blue was my connection to the source of magic within me, to my wildest, most true self.

In many ways, I began the journey of retrieving fragmented or lost aspects of my soul at the age of twenty-seven when I united with Blue. To support his healing, I massaged essential oils into his legs, practiced energy healing, and fed him anti-inflammatory supplements. We enjoyed long walks, both of us on foot. I'd tell him aloud that he was healed and strong. Within six months, we were galloping along the trails of Topanga Canyon's state park. We shared an exquisite bond based on deep trust, respect, and friendship. I rode him bareback and without a bit in his mouth, a way of riding based on a methodology called natural horsemanship that emphasizes fostering a trusting relationship with the horse rather than forcing the horse into submission. The term "breaking a horse" that is used to describe training epitomizes the patriarchal concept of domination over nature. It's about breaking the spirit rather than honoring and seeing the horse in his majesty and individuality, and cocreating in a symbiotic relationship. Blue and I spent nine glorious years together living in three different states. He was by my side through two significant relationships of my twenties and early thirties prior to meeting my husband and with me through the first two years of our marriage.

On this sweltering fall day, I was by his side all afternoon and into the night, praying my heart out and singing to him, begging Goddess not to take him from me. During this time, I began to hyperventilate, something I would go in and out of for the next week. After two vet visits to the barn, we trailered Blue to the animal hospital. Feeling hopeful once he was there, around 1:00 a.m., the vet techs convinced me to go home to try to sleep.

At 3:00 a.m., I received a phone call from the vet saying that Blue was getting worse and surgery wasn't an option. Blue was really suffering and must be euthanized. Frantic, I yelled, "Don't do anything until I get there!" and after hanging up screamed from the depths of my primal self, guttural screams that bellowed out of me as I dropped to my knees in grief, rage, and dread. I had never before experienced such intense and terrifying sounds coming out of me. I called my dad, and when I heard his voice on the line, I could barely form words.

"It's Blue," I said as I struggled for breath.

"You have to be strong for Blue," my dad said. "You only get to do this once. Conjure up all the love you feel for Blue and turn it into strength; that's what he needs now."

When I got to the hospital, I shared tender moments, gratitude, and loving final touch with my beloved companion who will always stay with me. I pressed my forehead to his, as we had done so many times before. I'd always felt an activation between the star on his forehead and my third eye. *He was my physical-world representation of everything magical.* I sang to him gently, telling him how deeply I will always love him. My beloved unicorn, my spirit twin, my best friend.

INANNA'S DESCENT

Gate 2: Removal of Her Lapis Necklace: My Magical Nature

As I walk through the second gate of the underworld, I am stripped of my connection to my truest self, my wild magical nature, my inner child, my Blue. I am so lost and alone.

At the second gate of the underworld, Inanna is asked to remove the small strand of lapis beads from her neck. Lapis lazuli is an ancient gemstone associated with the psychic center of the third eye, which governs perception and vision.

When Inanna asks the gatekeeper, "Why are you doing this?" she is told, "Silence, Inanna, the ways of the underworld are perfect.

They may not be questioned." *Inanna and I are both stripped of our most precious conduit to our inner vision, wisdom, and connection.*

Blue crossed the rainbow bridge early in the morning on October 25. While I was proud of the way I'd shown up and held space for him, I was absolutely devastated and beside myself with grief. Grieving all the visions of the future I held for Blue and me—him with my future children, him living with me at my home, all things that now could never be—I cried and cried, the flood of grief and sadness pouring through me. This was beyond anything I had ever felt before. I did not know how I would go on.

TEXT TO A FRIEND, OCTOBER 26, THE DAY AFTER BLUE'S PASSING

Yesterday was the biggest and most intense emotional release of my life, and I am delirious and exhausted. I screamed and cried until the point of convulsing. I couldn't stop my body from shaking in response to this loss. Ryan is afraid and doesn't know what to do with me; he's been calling my mom. I just need space to cry. I'm also doing so much shadow work with my priestess training. Serious purging is happening for me and such intense gripping fears and painful memories are coming forward.

PRIESTESS TRAINING

I could barely get myself to the airport to fly to Glastonbury a few days later, where I was to begin my second year of training. On the plane, the familiar pangs of sadness and grief ached in my chest, and I held my hand to my heart to self-soothe. *Ouch, what is that?* To my surprise, I felt a lump over my left breast, near my heart. It hurt and felt like a swollen spider bite. Feelings of panic raced through my mind at the thought of having a lump in my breast. *It must be a manifestation of grief after the traumatic loss I have been through. It will go away.*

I continued to feel the lump during the two weeks that followed in England and did my best to not think about it. It was my first time bringing my husband, Ryan, with me to Glastonbury, and I was so grateful to have him there. Walking through the fall landscape, leaves crunching beneath my feet, I often fell to my knees in tears. More than once I lay in full prostration, belly and heart melting into the ground, cupping the sides of my mouth and screaming down into the depths, giving my pain to Mother Earth to be transmuted.

When we returned home to California, I asked Ryan to feel the bump on my chest one more time. He had been telling me I was a hypochondriac and that it was one of my rib bones.

"But if it will make you feel better, go have it checked," he said.

The next day, I went to see a nearby gynecologist. My longtime doctor was two hours away in Los Angeles; we were living in Encinitas in north San Diego County. The gynecologist felt my breast and immediately sent me for a mammogram and ultrasound, possibly a biopsy. I was shocked. I had never had a mammogram; I was thirty-six. *You're not even supposed to get a mammogram until you're forty,* I thought. I was terrified yet desperately grasping to the belief this was all a mistake. *Clearly this is a manifestation of my grief.*

Changing into the pink gown for the mammogram, I looked around at the cold, sterile, uncomfortable atmosphere, all completely foreign territory for me and my lifestyle. I thought this feeling of unfamiliarity was a confirmation of the mistake that this all clearly was. *This is not my life.*

The mammogram really hurt, and the pressure of the ultrasound wand hurt even more. I clenched my fists and struggled for breath, asking the technician to please give me breaks. We shared uncomfortable silence as I asked her if she could tell what it was and she reminded me she's not allowed to say anything.

That night, the results came in as a level 5 (on a scale of 1–5), stating a high level of concern for malignancy and urging immediate biopsy. My system went into complete shock. I was trembling and unable to fully comprehend what was happening.

I reached out to a small group of dear friends and was comforted hearing things like, "Doctors are wrong all the time." *Yes, they are!* I thought. *I can't wait to get this over with and prove them wrong.* Grasping tightly to this notion with all I had, a text came in from a very dear and wise friend: "You are being asked to walk a very particular shadow path right now, my sister, one we may not understand for some time. Know that I am with you, I love you deeply, and I will walk with you every step of the way."

Something in me knew at this moment that I had cancer.

Journal Entry, One Week before Going to the Doctor

Dark goddess Keridwen came to me and I saw her in her beauty and profound loving. I saw how she is here for me, drumming, rattling, holding a sacred container. She is rubbing my back and making me healing brews. She's helping me release grief and ghosts from within to support my healing and transformation. She loves me deeply. She is not to be feared.

JOURNAL PROMPT

Who or what in your life helps you connect with your inner magic? Do you feel connected to your inner vision? Do you allow yourself to dream?

MEDITATION

Sit comfortably with your spine straight, or lie down, where you will not be disturbed.

Close your eyes, and begin taking in deep diaphragmatic breaths, in through the nose, filling and expanding the belly, and out through the mouth with an audible exhale...ahhh. Repeat three times.

Bring your awareness to the center of your forehead, the energy center of your third eye. Once you have focused your attention there, feel an indigo-colored energy expanding into the center of your head. Breathe in and out through your nose while maintaining internal focus in the space just behind the center of your forehead.

This is your center of vision, dreams, and imagination.

Ask inside to call forward the imagination of your inner child.

What did they daydream about? What fantastical worlds existed in the kingdom or queendom of their inner realm?

When in your life did you stop imagining this way?

At what age did you feel a loss of the innocent wonderment of childhood (for example, believing in Santa Claus or the tooth fairy)?

Call forward an image of yourself at this age. Trust yourself; your unconscious will bring forward the information needed, whether it comes in an image, memory, or feeling.

Imagine that your inner child is standing hand in hand with Inanna, and together, they are crossing the threshold through the second gate of the underworld.

There is nothing to fear, for your inner child holds the key to your inner sense of magic and wonder and is now on their way to retrieving something for you.

Watch them walk away and send them love.

When you are ready, bring your awareness back to the indigo-colored energy in the center of your head, emanating out through your brow.

Breathe deeply, allowing any feelings or sensations this process brought forward to arise.

Gently place your hands on your body, applying self-love and compassion.

When you are ready, open your eyes and journal any insights that came forward.

Blessed be.

Chapter Three

IDENTIFYING THE SPIRITUAL OPPORTUNITY

THIRD GATE: SILENCE

"The price of our vitality is the sum of all our fears."

~ David Whyte

IT'S CANCER

On December 1, I passed through the third gate of the underworld when I heard the words on the other end of the phone, "It's cancer." The most unbearable part of the initial news is that the presence of cancer is confirmed without knowing the stage, grade, or any further information. For the longest week of my life, I was haunted with thoughts like, "What if they tell me I have three weeks to live?"

On December 7, I met with my doctor, breast surgeon Kristi Funk, for the first time. She asked me if I wanted to have children, and if so, what day I was on in my menstrual cycle. For the previous two years, my husband and I had been actively trying to conceive. I had been reading fertility books, eating a fertility diet, doing preconception meditations, lying on the bed with my legs up the wall after making love, getting acupuncture every week, taking daily fertility herbs, and writing letters to the soul of my baby. The idea that having cancer could interfere with the possibility of becoming a mother was more than my system could process in the midst of the profound shock and trauma I was already coping with.

"Absolutely yes, I want to have children," I said. "I am on day twenty of my cycle."

Because of the invasive nature of the dis-ease, Dr. Funk said day twenty was perfect. The stimulation of hormones required for fertility treatment is not ideal for someone experiencing a hormone-driven cancer, which is what breast cancer is. Day twenty was perfect because the fertility treatment would start on the first or second day of bleeding, in approximately eight days. Had I been on day five, she would not have wanted to wait a month, because she felt it was urgent I begin chemo right away. "If you want to do a round of egg retrieval, you'll have to do it this cycle," she said. "I have a great doctor; I'll text her now."

For the next week, Ryan and I felt like we were being evacuated from our home in the midst of a natural disaster as we tried to navigate the torrential storm of emotions, panic, and anxiety as we simultaneously packed up what we needed from our home in Encinitas for Los Angeles for an unknown amount of time. As we faced what we knew would be incredible hardship, we decided to move to Los Angeles indefinitely, where we would be surrounded by the support of dear friends and family while receiving the best medical care. We needed to find a place to stay with our two cats before I began fertility treatment. The hormone stimulation would begin right away, the egg retrieval surgery was estimated to occur around Christmas, and I would begin chemo January 2.

This was the darkest time of my life. I was in shock, flooded with tears, rage, despair, grief, and the deepest spiritual pain and heartache. I went in daily for ultrasounds and blood draws while giving myself several injections a day over my womb. All the while, I tried to process the fact that I had cancer and would be going through chemo in a few weeks. I was in a hurricane of emotions, sometimes lying on the floor crying uncontrollably for hours. The hormone fluctuations I was experiencing with the fertility treatments added to the swirling feelings of complete loss of control.

My close friend April, who is a shaman, told me the night of my diagnosis that facing death is a shamanic initiation. I felt in my bones that Goddess was initiating me into something, a deep power or truth, and remembered the words I spoke in my dedication, asking to become Her clear channel.

One day, as I lay crying on the floor, imagining my body being poisoned by chemo, my husband said to me, "Sweetheart, this is going to save your life. You have so many skills. I think you need to try to see the chemo as sacred medicine that your body needs."

A light bulb went off inside me, and I felt hope for the first time. I knew I could make this beautiful. I spoke to one of my friends about creating a new name for breast cancer, something I had done in the past for clients. For example, a client with polycystic ovary syndrome (PCOS) playfully renamed it "pure creative ovaries singing." Renaming things takes the power away from the fear associated with the dis-ease or condition and turns it into something else of your creation. Using the letters BC, my friend Bonne and I came up with "beaming cellular cooperation," visualizing all my cells restructuring themselves in perfect harmony, balance, and radiant health. I made a vision board with Louise Hay affirmations and wrote my new name for breast cancer at the center. I lit a candle in front of it and took a photo, making it the screen saver on my phone.

Even though I loved my new term for my visualizations, I noticed

I would say "the C word" rather than "beaming cellular cooperation" when I spoke. One day, Ryan referred to it as "critters," and that
really stuck. I liked calling it critters because, for me, this completely
took the power away from the stigma associated with the word cancer. A critter sounds like a temporary annoyance that you could flick
away with your finger, and this is exactly what I planned to do.

Louise Hay's book *You Can Heal Your Life* is one I reference regularly to gain insight into the underlying causes of physical ailments.
I looked up her affirmations for breasts, cancer, and breast problems, and I spoke these affirmations every day, creating a recording
of myself that I listened to often. There is something very powerful
about listening to your own voice. There is soul medicine in it, just
as there is soul medicine in gazing lovingly into your own eyes while
speaking affirmations into a mirror.

HEALING: WESTERN MEDICINE

At the time of diagnosis, I had a negative view of Western medicine
and had always treated myself holistically. I used homeopathy, acupuncture, supplements, and herbal remedies. I drank healing ton-
ics and superfood smoothies. I ate only organic food. I had been a
vegetarian for a decade. I worked with crystals, vibrational healing,
and visualization. I was completely unfamiliar with the construct of
medicine into which I was being thrust. I felt I was being forcefully
catapulted like a cannonball into a place of complete unknown, both
within myself and in my external environment.

In all of my experiences with therapy, emotional healing, and plant
medicine journeys, in which the aim was to access repressed emotions and pain from my unconscious, I had never come close to the
depth of pain and despair I was living with now. Before hearing the
words, "You have cancer," I was playfully standing on the shores, letting the waves wash over my feet while remaining comfortable in my

life. After those words were spoken, I was plunged into the deepest, darkest, coldest uninhabited waters of the ocean with no oxygen tank. Grappling with the idea of filling my body with poison was beyond belief. I was so angry.

I was beginning to understand the nature of my diagnosis, which was about a five-centimeter span of ductal carcinoma in situ (DCIS) with three invasive ductal carcinoma tumors, which spread into my lymph nodes. While ductal carcinoma is contained within a milk duct, invasive carcinoma means it has broken beyond the duct wall and spread. It was stage 3.

At first, I feared that cancer spread through the lymph system, although I later learned that it spreads through the blood. Once the presence of a tumor is in your body, at any stage, there are circulating tumor cells traveling around your bloodstream looking for another home. The doctors told me chemo was necessary to eradicate those circulating cells. A resounding truth from deep in my bones told me right away that I had to do it.

As clear as this knowing was, it was very difficult for me to accept. In the alternative-minded spiritual community I was part of, people didn't do chemo. Juicing wheatgrass, raw food diets, and Rick Simpson's cannabis oil were modalities that felt more socially acceptable. A small part of me feared I needed to prove myself as a healer—that I could heal myself from anything. *Was Western medicine a cop-out?*

Regardless of the methods I chose, I was staring directly into the face of a terrifying beast, with eyes as doorways into the black void that took the place of my own power. Chung Fu, one of my group of alternative healers, explained that, although cancer is silent, chemo shows you how powerful it is because it matches the cancer in its power. He told me that the most important thing for me was to make all choices from deep within. This was my healing journey. I needed to trust myself and not be swayed by the opinions of others. My life depended on it.

HEALERS ALONG THE WAY

Chung Fu

I first heard about Chung Fu from a friend in the goddess community. She shared about her work with him one afternoon over tea after I asked about an image framed on her altar, a beautiful painting of an old Chinese sage that emanated kindness and wisdom.

"That's Chung Fu," she said. "He guides and supports many of the women in the priestess community."

I felt a stirring from within and knew right away I had been divinely guided to work with this ascended being and spirit guide, and his trance medium, Sally Pullinger. I experienced my first session with him just three months before being diagnosed. Even though Sally, as the vehicle through which Chung Fu communicates, is a woman, Chung Fu is a male presence. Sitting before Sally and witnessing her enter a state of trance is a holy experience. Tears often spill over my cheeks as I feel the presence of Spirit palpably enter the room.

When I received the news that I was facing cancer, I immediately reached out to the Pullinger family, who live in Avalon together as a tribe, unified in sacred healing work. I was so grateful they made time for me to connect with Chung Fu over the phone the very next day.

Session with Chung Fu, December 9, Just after Receiving Diagnosis

I begin by saying I'm very committed to the inner work, to clearing and releasing the ancestral karma, letting go of whatever I need to. I'm open to anything. I know this is a very deep part of my soul's journey.

Chung Fu: That's right, it's a journey and the strength and spirit to do the work that's required of you will rise up from inside you. The only absolute rule is not to suppress anything. Cancer is a dis-ease of suppression; it stems from absence and fear. Part of you is not present because you were forced to suppress your feelings for one reason or another when you were younger and couldn't get the words out, or didn't know how to express yourself. After that, you were afraid to upset the apple cart. You didn't want to hurt people. And you got into a habit of suppression. And then, your body became angry and called out, "Why aren't you shouting? I'm angry. Why aren't you saying it?"

And when you didn't respond, your body acquiesced, gave in, saying, "Well alright, I'll put my anger away again, then."

And in those places, the real you couldn't be present because you were basically pretending; you were not in your truth. When you suppress emotion, and when emotion suppression becomes habitual, the absence is created. You're not really present. So, your meditations, and your inner practices, have to be about calling for emotional authenticity. Calling for presence, for your power to be present, as you truly are. To say things as they are, to own your feelings, to speak them. As you go through this journey, the people in your life might need a bit of warning: "I'm warning you, my dear friend, who slightly irritates me, to whom I've been agreeable all my life. I'm warning you that I may not behave with my normal peace, and calm. I may get a bit irritable, and it's just my condition."

While what you know, for yourself, is that you're just letting yourself discharge emotion as it comes up. You must change your habits.

"Yes," I replied. "I'm honestly grateful for the opportunity to change this deeply ingrained habit of people-pleasing. And smiling, and holding things back. Or always saying things in the 'nicest' way. I can think of so many times I swallowed my feelings, or my truth. Or said something in a passive way instead of directly. Or said half of what I wanted to say, and was left with the residue inside to fester, unspoken."

Chung Fu explained that cancer represents a place inside that has been abandoned, a place where I was no longer inhabiting my truth. He described my diagnosis as a call for presence and authenticity, and said it was critical for me to discharge my emotions and *"let it all out."* He said there's a massive emotional underbelly to any cancer experience and that it was vital for me to express my needs and *"say it like it is"* truthfully and authentically.

You can still be polite and say it like it is.

This resonated with me, as I had suffered for years with fear and avoidance of confrontation, which often meant I avoided speaking up for myself or fully expressing my opinion. He said that sometimes screaming was essential to release this suppression. I remembered my guttural screaming that began the night I lost Blue and the cathartic screaming that had continued for the month between then and now. Chung Fu said actually hearing the sound and power in my voice was important, as this would empower me.

The screaming was hard for my husband to hear and part of me felt I needed to contain it to make him feel better. But that behavior would fall into the people-pleasing category, which was no longer permitted. Screaming felt good, natural, and exactly what my body needed to do instinctively. My body trembled and shook as I wept, and a fire rose in my chest and erupted from my throat, like a volcano of primal rage.

To support my emotional body in riding these waves, Chung Fu suggested a Bach flower essence for shock, called Star of Bethlehem, which was massively supportive in soothing me and calming my nervous system. I also started taking the Bach flower essence Aspen for stress and anxiety, as well as Rescue Remedy. I took these constantly, and they provided great relief.

Michael Hayes

During my time at USM, I met Alisha and Michael Hayes, two incredibly spiritually attuned and gifted healers. Michael supported many of the students at USM in healing wounds that had carried over from previous lifetimes and clearing karma. In the classroom, if someone was processing something they just couldn't get to the bottom of or expressing a level of emotion that didn't seem sensible related to the issue at hand, at a certain point our teachers would say, "I would suggest going to see Michael Hayes."

I knew immediately that I wanted to talk to Michael about my diagnosis and what was going on with me spiritually. I also knew I needed one session with him, and after that, I needed to work with Alisha. I had met Alisha a few times and felt drawn to her soft, angelic presence and palpable strength and depth.

Michael told me that *cancer is best perceived as a teacher.* It had come into my life to teach me and help me heal. Often, this dis-ease stems from "a wish to not feel so much," and what's underneath it is, "I feel too much, too hard, too intensely." The dis-ease comes from trying to pull back from the intensity of living, so on a deep level, it's an antilife choice. Shifts in energy flow follow that choice and create the physical manifestation of the dis-ease. In working with me, he saw something around age fourteen that triggered a karma in which I chose to go against my abilities—to be less than I am—as a survival choice, a type of self-denial and self-betrayal. He was also feeling a karma from another life in which I didn't want to be burned at the stake, and I pretended to be like everyone else rather than express my truth. He said this, too, was a choice of self-denial and self-betrayal, and when everything happened at age fourteen that made me shut down, that karma was activated because I was denying myself. The opportunity and the healing are in forgiving the self-judgment about pulling back from who I am, for trying to belong, and for trying to please others.

I forgive myself for judging myself for pulling back from who I am.

I forgive myself for judging myself as trying to belong.

I forgive myself for judging myself as trying to please others.

I forgive myself for judging myself for denying my truth to please others.

The opportunity is to let go of these judgments—from this lifetime or any other—and free myself of being trapped in self-denial and in the rigid "either/or" misunderstanding that "I am who I am" or I'm *not*. He spoke about releasing the paradigm of either/or from my consciousness and shifting into the perspective of both/and, living into the essentialness of who I am, and adapting if need be. His example was about driving in England. When there, I don't drive on the right side of the road because that's the way I know how to drive. I adapt and drive on the left because that's the safest way to drive, not to mention what the law requires. I can still be true to the essentialness of who I am while driving on the left side of the road.

He affirmed my ability to read a person's energy and/or the energy of a room and feel what is appropriate to share. This doesn't mean that if I can't share everything I shut down and share nothing. It means not talking about quantum physics with someone in fifth grade. It's about adaptability. As he spoke about adaptability, I could make out the words "adapt or die" over his left shoulder on a vision board collage hanging on the wall behind him. Adapt *while being true to my essence*. There are different ways I can bring my energy forward while being true to my essence.

Michael gave me three pillars of wisdom to carry forward into my journey:

"**The first law of Spirit is acceptance.**" I needed to fully accept the situation I am in.

"**The second law of Spirit is cooperation.**" Work with cancer as a teacher, allow the work to guide me, and go willingly into the territory this requires.

"**The third law of Spirit is enthusiasm.**" I can wish things were different, but this is no time for bitterness. It's the time to bring my best self forward.

"Mastery is not about being above the conditions of the world," Michael said. "It's about how we relate to the conditions of the world. It's all about learning and growing."

He asked me where in my life I had been pretending. Where was I putting energy into something I didn't like? Was I buying into idealistic reasons for doing things instead of being in true joy? Where had I made compromises and gone along with things I didn't want to do? I thought of a few months prior when I had agreed to colead a retreat I had already been running on my own with a woman, Jin, with whom I didn't want to collaborate.

Jin was quite a bit older than I was, with a lot more teaching experience. I felt I *should* be honored that she wanted to work with me. I told myself this while everything in me screamed, "*No!*" I avoided the discomfort of turning her down by saying "yes" when I didn't mean it, a choice that pained me for months. I definitely knew what Michael was talking about.

"Why would you do something that doesn't align with who you are, or what you want, or make you feel good?" he asked.

Alisha Das

A couple weeks later, I had my first session with Alisha, and I knew instantly I had been led to the right place. I was stunned at the immediate alignment Alisha's assessment had with the wisdom of Chung Fu, as well as the way it mirrored the themes laid out by Michael. During our first session, Alisha homed in on key aspects of my personal history that she felt were imperative to my complete healing. The first two were healing the trauma that occurred around age fourteen and fifteen, and having the willingness to open my spiritual vision again. I have to admit this frightened me a bit. She said cancer takes about twenty years from the time of the wound or fragment in consciousness to manifest in the physical body. This timeline accurately pinpointed when I shut down my spiritual gifts as a teen.

I'M A WITCH BEING HUNTED

When I was fourteen, in my first year of boarding school in Colorado Springs, I offered past-life regressions to my friends, channeling one of my spirit guides whom I called Lionianisthma, or Li. My friends and I would huddle in my dorm room as my spirit guide spoke through me. Something about our nightly gatherings troubled our dorm parents and, for the first time in my life, I was pegged as a troublemaker. These dorm parents, also our teachers, were convinced that during our innocent spiritual explorations, we were actually plotting schemes to break the rules at school. Soon, there were rumors that I was casting spells and talking with ghosts, and my peers were afraid of me.

My friend Sabrina was the first person I'd ever met who was my age and shared my spiritual interests. We became friends when she told me she saw my rainbow aura with white around it, knowing that white meant I was attuned to the spiritual realms. She was magical, and I loved the bond I shared with her and two other friends.

Sabrina had gone through a terrible and traumatic experience of sexual assault by her teacher and guidance counselor, something this private boarding school would do anything to cover up. Shortly after this came out among the teaching staff, Sabrina and I were called individually to sit in front of the discipline committee. At boarding school, this punishment is referred to as "getting a DC." I walked into a room with about eight teachers looking quite intimidating and authoritarian, all sitting on the same side of a table facing the door with one empty chair across from them. As I took my seat, the headmaster stared down at me and said, "Students around campus are calling you a witch. What do you have to say about that?"

I felt an energy rise from deep within. I held his gaze as I calmly replied, "I *am* a witch."

He shuddered with fear, and I felt the immense power of what I had said. He expelled me from school and said I had twenty-four hours to pack up and leave campus. He said I was never allowed to step foot there again. He would notify my parents immediately.

The terror that seized my body was immense and all-consuming, and a shrill voice within me frantically urged, *"Run away as fast as you can! Run for the hills and don't look back!"* I feared my parents were going to literally kill me when they came to pick me up. This profoundly confused me and didn't make sense in my mind, but the imminent threat continued to erupt within me like electricity arcing through my body.

When my parents arrived, after driving six hours from Telluride, they didn't offer hugs or smiles. They clearly showed their disappointment in me and let me know I would not be happy at home. Before sending me to boarding school in ninth grade, they had lovingly reassured me that if I hated it, I could always come home. But when I did have a terrible time and cried hysterically on the pay phone begging them to let me come home, they wouldn't. Now, as we loaded my things into the car, they said, "You're going to a different boarding school. You have no choice now; you cannot come home. And you've *got* to stop telling people you're a witch!"

The extreme terror I experienced was something I had no skills to cope with and didn't understand for many years to come. Later, I would learn through deep shamanic work that this kind of terror and paralyzing fear that seizes the body is always from the past. It's from something that has indeed already happened, if not earlier in this life, in a previous incarnation. When it makes its presence known, this is an indication the trauma is ready to be seen and healed. On a soul level, my experience getting a DC was a familiar reenactment of trials I had been through in previous incarnations with much worse consequences. My opportunity would be to reclaim the power I lost in those previous experiences.

A PSYCHIATRIST AND RITALIN

Just before my experience with the discipline committee, the school sent me to see a psychiatrist. I always had a naturally serene disposition, yet suddenly I was diagnosed with attention-deficit/hyperactivity disorder and put on Ritalin, a terrible drug. My parents never questioned anything the school said and that was that. I was forced to take medication in front of the school nurse twice a day for the next four years (this carried over to my next school in Dobbs Ferry, New York).

This drug completely shut down my creativity, spiritual connection, sense of self, and capacity to feel emotions, especially happiness and laughter. I hated the feeling of Ritalin! I felt like a robot: blank, empty, and devoid of feeling. I loved the weekends because I felt my body. All through high school I lived for those two days when I came back to life. The sensation of laughing with my friends felt *so* good. The school in Colorado Springs had completely shut me down and systematically suppressed my true expression, creating a deep chasm and fragmentation within my psyche. Part of me left at age fifteen and didn't return for quite some time.

Alisha reiterated that cancer on the left side of my body meant it was related to my femininity and the lineage of my mother line, including my expression of feminine energy. The right side is related to masculine energy and the father line. Alisha is an intuitive healer, and every week, she looked at past-life scenarios that were underlying my present feelings to support me in healing at the deepest level available. In each session, I worked with compassionate self-forgiveness to forgive judgments I had placed on myself or others in current situations, as well as judgments from past-life scenarios. Doing this, I always experienced a release of immense pressure within my emotional body and heart, and felt lightness and clarity after.

Although I didn't know it when I reached out to her, Alisha had recently healed from her own bout with uterine cancer. She was the first person who mentioned the term "cancer personality" to me. As

Alisha explained, there is enough commonality among people who experience cancer that there has been psychological study into the personality traits cancer patients share. Given my background in spiritual psychology, I was not surprised to hear this and eager to know more. I learned about the traits, as stated by Dr. Douglas Brodie,[1] associated with cancer personality. A few of them immediately stood out to me:

"...exhibits a strong tendency toward carrying other people's burdens and toward taking on extra obligations, often 'worrying for others...'"

"...a deep-seated need to make others happy. Being a 'people pleaser' with a great need for approval..."

"...a long-standing tendency to suppress 'toxic emotions,' particularly anger."

I related to the themes represented in these traits: people-pleasing, taking on others' burdens, suppressing anger. I first understood the energetic dynamic around taking on others' burdens when I spoke to a brilliant medical intuitive, Laura Kamm, who said, "You do recognize that your nervous system is a highly responsive nervous system to other people's energies, the world, and the environment, right?"

She shared that I absorbed the energy of the world around me starting at a very young age, and by ten, I was completely overwhelmed. She said this took a toll on my nervous system, which in turn affected my endocrine system that responds to the signals of the nervous system. When I was put on Ritalin at age fifteen, this capped my effervescence; I wasn't able to experience the level of vitality I was capable of. It was as though my world went from vivid color to black and white. This changed my chemistry, which affected all the other systems in my body. It numbed out my nervous system to a degree that it shut down intuitive receptors. Understanding that

---

1   Brodie, Dr. Douglas, "Psycho-Oncology: Discover How Stress Causes Cancer" http://www.alternative-cancer-care.com/the-cancer-personality.html

I'm driven by a highly empathic nervous system, which is unique, helped me to understand more deeply the impact of taking on other people's burdens.

Chung Fu and Alisha had both instantly homed in on ages fourteen and fifteen, the need to heal the trauma that had separated me from my spiritual gifts and to heal karma with my mother. Chung Fu said that many aspects of my teen self were unmothered, and deep healing needed to occur in this area. After being expelled from the boarding school in Colorado Springs, I went across the country to Dobbs Ferry, New York, about a thirty-minute train ride from New York City. For the rest of high school, age fifteen to eighteen, my mother was physically absent the majority of the time.

Chung Fu spoke of the effect this had on me following the trauma and self-abandonment that resulted from my expulsion from school. I had abandoned what was truly aligned with my heart because I was scared of others condemning me. Going through the depression and inner isolation that followed, without receiving love and nurturing from my family, had created a hard shell around this teen aspect of myself that needed to be retrieved and healed. He and Alisha both zeroing in on this particular time in my life blew me away.

SESSION WITH CHUNG FU, DECEMBER 9, CONTINUED

Chung Fu: The level of stress that's alive in your culture means that you hardly need to do anything to be carrying stress. Stress emanates out of the very bones of the culture. It rolls off other people; it's there in the lifestyle. So yes, you've moved into your adult years becoming very aware of what's going on inside you, making big moves, of course, to develop and change. Today, I'd like you to go back and look at all of the factors that have led to this manifestation, this way of being you've learned, that is both emotional and ancestral. Start to listen to your inner child because the left breast is mother. The left breast is where there's a yearning, an unfulfilled need. There's a specific place—you can feel it; probably as I say this, it slightly aches.

Once again, I nod in assent as Chung Fu seems to know exactly what I'm feeling.

Pay attention to your discomfort because it's talking to you. Cancer is very alive and like you, as a living thing, cancer can grow. Once it has established itself, it has a lot of power. It has taken up residence in a place where you lacked your own power. This place of need and emptiness is an unfulfilled absence. It's a part of you that's trying to come in, arrive—trying to be the mother you didn't have, though she's always done her very best. However, something here is very clear: an anger toward your mother. This is because the nurturing she offered you wasn't exactly right for you, however well-intentioned. There was something missing in her emotional approach to you.

MY MOTHER WOUND

This is a wound many of us have. Although I knew it was true, it was hard for me to completely acknowledge it because I love my mother. I see how my needs hadn't been met, especially in the years I was sent away to boarding school, yet I also see how she did the best she could at the time with the skills and awareness she had. My mother wound had nothing to do with the amount of love I have for my mother. It didn't make her wrong or bad, and ultimately, it didn't even have anything to do with her. It was about me and the wounding that occurred within me as a result of the circumstances of my adolescence. It was the emotion that lived within me without relief that had festered.

Being sent away to boarding school was traumatic. Even though I had wonderful friends, being across the country from my family and visiting home three times over ten months from ages fourteen to eighteen was extremely difficult. When summer rolled around, there was always an awkward adjustment to actually being at home. *Do I have rules? A curfew?* I didn't know how to relate to things that were part of most teens' daily lives.

I remember eating magic mushrooms once over a school break in Colorado and being overwhelmed by a longing to feel at home. When I thought of home, I pictured the dorm room I shared with my dear friend Kym, and the construction paper stars we had cut from many colors and stuck all over the ceiling. It struck me that technically, at that moment, I was home in Telluride; however, when I tried to connect with the feeling of home, I saw only the dorm.

My mother also has a mother wound and felt she hadn't received love from her mother in the way she needed. It's a generational pattern that ultimately goes back to our perceived separation from Source, or divine nature, and wanting to return to that feeling of supreme mother love from Goddess. Perhaps this is why mother and daughter wounds are as they are; mothers and daughters all collectively carry a piece of the deep wound of the divine feminine being eliminated from our culture for thousands of years. Most human beings experience a sense of separation from the Divine when they pass through the veil and come into this incarnation. Maybe this is exacerbated in women due to the lack of acknowledgement of the Goddess in our Western world, and this disconnect manifests as the mother wound.

The connection we have with our mothers is in our blood. I came from my mother's body, and was born of her blood, the waters of her womb. When I was in my mother's womb, I was imprinted with her energy and traces of my grandmother's energy, as well. All ova that will eventually become eggs when a woman reaches maturity are formed in utero. So, the egg that was impregnated by my father's sperm that became the embryo that ultimately became me, came into being in my grandmother's womb when my mother was a fetus. The womb is the connection to the ancestral mother line back to the womb of creation. The blood is imprinted with the memories of how all the women in this line have or have not been loved. Some say there are seven generations of ancestral patterns imprinted on us while in the womb. My mother wound is an ancestral mother wound, one that my mother passed to me and didn't consciously know she had. She knew she hadn't received love from her mother as a child, and she, too, had been sent away to boarding school at age fourteen. She wasn't aware of the inherited wound until I spoke to her about it after my mastectomy surgery. Perhaps healing these deep spiritual and emotional wounds requires the shedding of physical blood. Perhaps this happens when we've arrived at the source of the wound—it's bloody.

As I marveled at the undeniable truth in the wounds being revealed to me, I recalled my first session with Chung Fu, which was three months *before* the cancer diagnosis, and just days before my first priestess dedication on the autumnal equinox—the ceremony I awoke from with overwhelming dread.

SESSION WITH CHUNG FU, THREE MONTHS BEFORE DIAGNOSIS

Chung Fu: You bring a lot of presence with you, beloved. I think you do a lot of work with Spirit, don't you?

I replied that I did, but didn't elaborate because with Chung Fu's insight, it didn't seem necessary.

There are a lot of beings here. You're a channel yourself.

I had a feeling he would talk about that, although this was something, at the time, I hadn't done any healing work around. I shared that I began channeling when I was thirteen. I'd lie down on the floor of the library and channel my spirit guide for friends at school. I mention that I was punished at a young age for that and felt that I had closed this part of myself off.

Let's talk about this time of your life and what you're experiencing in general so that we can see how to help you open these doors. They are already open at certain levels, but I can see that's not something you're experiencing in your mental, emotional, and physical world. So, what's filling up your world? Let's have a look at what's in the way and talk to that small place in you. Let's convince her that you're not going to get punished for it this time. You came to see me, so clearly, you're in a place in your life where you're willing to talk to Spirit.

You're moving into a much wilder area, the priestess area of your being, and it's full of all sorts of pain. I'm sure you have found some of it already. Places where you were definitely shut down and where you're having to reclaim a deep part of your soul. This is going to continue as you go deeper. You will get there, beloved; it's happening. You're doing it. The energy is definitely moving. It's a bit like an earthquake rumbling away and the cracks are appearing. You're very aware of the depths of your being. It's alright; I don't have a worry about it. You're going to progress along this path and Goddess Herself will shake you up from inside—in the beauty way, and sometimes, in a very scary way in terms of what comes up to be met, but it's alright. You've found support; you've found a way to grow, and that's wonderful. What you must make sure of is that you remain authentic, that people know you; don't hide your transformation.
"Don't hide who I am?"

That's right. This is an old paradigm—the sisters that hide because they're afraid of jealousy or being put down by other sisters. In the community of sisters, go gently; don't run before you can walk, but hold yourself as the spirit you truly are and take your rightful place.

Sometimes that's difficult because you're shining a bit brighter, or you know a bit more, or you're just a bit wiser, but the other person is a bit more something else.

The sisterhood work is in its initiatory phases; it's quite new all over the world. Women waking up to the fact of how terribly they've been triggered into competition and betrayal of each other, and not knowing how to support and empower each other because there are few models in the outer world. All these things need to be understood and worked with, and I think you're doing very well, although you're still doing the classic thing of hiding, but that's alright right now. You're moving.

Looking back, I see the foreshadowing of an intense initiatory journey of Goddess shaking me from the inside. At the third gate of the underworld, Goddess shook me from my throat, stripping me of the habitual pattern of keeping quiet, of not expressing my authentic self. The words spoken to me, "You have cancer," changed the trajectory of my life in profound ways, and I would never be the same. I no longer had the option of hiding from my soul's true expression or the false sense of safety I received from hiding.

INANNA'S DESCENT

Gate 3: Stripped of Her Beads: Silence

Inanna enters the third gate of the underworld, where she is stripped of the beads hanging around her neck, at her throat chakra. The throat chakra is the center of communication and expression. She is stripped of the power of her words, of the power to express authority over her life as queen of heaven. As she moves further into the underworld, she is stripped of the control she believes she possesses over her life. She is pulled into a realm where none of the rules or reference points of the upperworld apply, into the complete unknown, with no familiar methods of communication.

Words spoken by others that I had believed to be true, and words I had withheld, were forcefully ripped from the walls of my throat, where they had petrified like stone—all the times I hadn't spoken up for myself, that I swallowed my feelings, that I felt intimidated or afraid to ask a question, or repressed communication. As I walk through the third gate of the underworld, I am stripped of the option to remain silent in my life, stripped of the perceived safety I believed I was granted by withholding my authentic expression. Goddess was teaching me that I could no longer live this way.

. . .

The loss of control that I felt when the words "You have cancer" were spoken to me shattered me into a million pieces. Ideas about the life I would lead, the children and grandchildren I would have, any possibility of the future I felt was available for me, had been ripped away. I was standing on a barren wasteland of fear and powerlessness, with no words or familiar methods of communication. I was in the complete unknown. Deep inside, I knew this teacher—cancer—had shown up in my life for a reason. For me to heal fully, I needed to listen to what she had to teach.

Journal Entry

Priestess sister Graell came to visit and we were sharing about my healing journey; how Goddess is working through me to dismantle all that's been in the way of my experiencing Her purely, so that I may truly know Her within my body. Graell looked at me with a smile and said, "Cancer. Can—C—Her." This was a eureka moment for me! Can See Her.

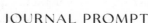

JOURNAL PROMPT

When in your life have you stayed silent about something meaningful to you? When or with whom do you suppress your truth? Do you have fear of authentically expressing yourself?

MEDITATION

Sit comfortably with your spine straight, or lie down, where you will not be disturbed.

Close your eyes, and begin taking in deep diaphragmatic breaths, in through the nose, filling and expanding the belly, and out through the mouth with an audible exhale...ahhh. Repeat three times.

Imagine an elevator in your mind's eye. As the doors open, you step inside.

The elevator begins moving down from the center of your head, through your neck, where it stops in your throat.

The doors open and you step outside into your throat chakra, the energy center that rules all forms of communication and emanates the color blue.

With your awareness fully present within this energy center, take a moment to notice the terrain. What is the quality of energy present? Does it feel stuck, hard, prickly? Or does it feel relaxed and open? Does it feel warm or cool? Allow yourself to experience the sensations here.

Now it's time to go deeper. Ask yourself: What words have been held within these sensations? What has been left unexpressed? What messages did you tell yourself at the time you withheld these words?

Give yourself permission to allow any memories to come forward, meeting them with compassion for yourself.

See Inanna standing before you, at the entrance to the third gate of the underworld. She asks you to visualize an object that represents these unspoken words.

When you are ready, she extends her hands in an inviting gesture and this object is expelled from your throat. As you gaze upon this object in Inanna's hands, allow yourself to release sound from your throat. Give yourself permission to express any sound that is present to release, whether it's a moan, groan, sigh, scream, a tone, or spoken words. If words are present, speak out the words that were withheld in the past, giving this stuck energy an opportunity to be jostled loose and set free. Guided by the sound of your voice, Inanna steps across the third gate of the underworld, carrying the object that was expelled from your throat with her. She is supporting you in releasing what has held you back from authentic expression.

Take a deep breath and lovingly place your hands on your throat, filling this center with your love. Imagine a person or an animal whom you love unconditionally, and send the loving you feel for that being into your throat center now.

When you are ready, open your eyes and journal any insights that came forward.

Blessed be.

Chapter Four

WHY NOT "FUCK CANCER"?

FOURTH GATE: WITHHOLDING LOVE

"Out beyond ideas of wrongdoing and right-doing,
there is a field, I'll meet you there."

~ Rumi

Whenever I see #fuckcancer, it makes me cringe. The idea of creating a "war" within my body to "beat" cancer is the opposite of my nature. I don't resonate with the attitude of turning against my body, especially while my body and I are in crisis and seeking healing. Cancer is serious, absolutely; it's terrifying. But I believe that illness is a way the soul speaks through the body, urgently calling out for healing in a certain area. I felt there was an unseen wound within me that created the condition—and not from a place of weakness. *I'm not to blame for the cancer* that appeared in my body. Thoughts that I'm somehow guilty of harming myself and could have prevented the cancer from happening are not my perspective. I believe that within the construct of my mind, body, emotions, unconscious, and spirit, there was an *opening* in my consciousness that allowed this dis-ease to manifest *because it has something to teach me.*

Some of you are with me, but for others, this may be a hard place to follow. Cancer is such an individualized thing; every person's cancer puzzle is completely their own, and the causes aren't exactly the same for everyone. I believe there are many different factors that contribute to cancer manifesting in the body, including the stresses in life and *how we relate to stress*, our emotional state and the way we express or deny these emotions, the environmental toxins we encounter and toxic buildup in the body, the spiritual lessons each of us has come to learn in this lifetime, and the evolution of our soul. Healing is complex, multidimensional, and completely unique to the individual. What works for one person may not work for another.

I knew deep down when I was diagnosed that to fully heal and eradicate the dis-ease from my body and consciousness, I had to embrace my situation and love myself—all of me, *especially* my left breast. I had to enter into a dialogue with cancer. Why was it here? What had it come to teach me? How could I fully heal whatever it was here to show me so that it would leave and never come back again? The attitude of saying "fuck you" to my body felt so harsh, as though there was an aspect of me I wanted to beat up. The "fuck cancer" perspective wants to blame, judge, and fight with reality to make the experience wrong. I believe to heal a situation we must fully accept it as it is to begin the process. I needed to do the work to accept the formidable diagnosis of cancer as my first step toward healing.

Embracing and loving what is, however, does not mean approving of it or justifying it. It means being gentle and nurturing myself and being fully present in the now. It means not making my body wrong or buying into the misunderstanding that I must have done something wrong for this to happen. My body needs to be my best friend and biggest ally in this journey, and we need to heal together.

Cancer is becoming rampant in our society, and although that is frightening, how might things change if we start to listen to what it's trying to teach us? I am reminded of my favorite Rumi quote: "Out beyond ideas of wrongdoing and right-doing there is a field. I'll meet you there." That's how I felt about cancer. I would meet it in Rumi's field. And I was pretty sure that out there in Rumi's field, I would find a group of sacred friends who would be brave enough and love me enough to walk the journey with me.

INNER HEALING

Prayer Circle

The prayer circle I created for myself was a lifeline. I experienced an aha moment of clarity when I first sat down to write out the list of women I really desired to be with me in my prayer circle. This was not the list of women I felt obligated to include because their feelings might be hurt if they weren't asked. Before cancer, I definitely would have made the list based on this criteria. I had always tried to micromanage situations so no one's feelings would be hurt, or so that, most importantly, I could *avoid confrontation* at all costs. As I wrote the list of women in my ideal prayer circle, I remembered one of my mantras from Alisha: "Everything I am doing is *for* me and my healing, not *against* anyone else." Fifteen wonderful women responded with an enthusiastic yes, and my own unique prayer circle was born.

EMAIL INVITATION TO FIFTEEN FRIENDS

Hello, my loves,

It has been suggested by one of my teachers that I create a daily prayer circle with an intimate group of friends. One of my sisters in Glaston-bury is going through her own journey with cancer and her dear friends created a similar prayer group for her. I am deeply inspired and moved by the power those involved are experiencing.

The idea is based on Lynne McTaggart's book The Power of Eight, which describes the miracles that occur when small groups gather to focus on a collective intention. Chung Fu shared that as I am in this powerful experience of initiation, all of those in the field of energy with me will experience their own transformation and healing. My friend who is moving through her own cancer journey said that the friends sending her prayers and energy were having incredible healings of their own.

So, here is what I am asking from the depth of my heart...

I would like to set a time twice a day for everyone to tune in over the ethers and send a specific healing prayer or visualization out to me for ten minutes. For example, at 8:30 a.m. and 9:30 p.m. It's okay if only once a day works for you, however, it's best to have as much energy gathered at one time as possible. Some sisters are on the East Coast, so the evening times may not work for everyone. My friend suggested that in certain circumstances, if someone can't tune in at the specific time, they send their prayer earlier and "intend it forward" by sending it ahead to join the group energy at the specific time.

If you feel called to dive into this, I will share more of my personal experiences right now—what this healing journey is for me and specific visuals I would love for you to help me hold. We can create a What's App group where we can share experiences and visions that come forward during the prayers, and where I can check in via voice memo and share what's happening for me. I can let the group know if I desire extra support around anything specific that comes up for me.

I realize there is a deepening occurring in my personal acceptance of my situation—that I have cancer and that I need help. My intention is to heal everything in my consciousness that created this circumstance so that I eradicate this condition from my system forever!

I have been receiving so much beautiful support from my light infusion team—April, Keri, and Val—and on the days I receive infusions, I also receive an abundance of beautiful prayers from all of you, my gorgeous and amazing sisters. Those days have been profoundly healing and powerful. I have noticed that after that, as the effects of the chemo kick in, I really struggle, especially the first week. When I'm exhausted and in bed all day, the best I can do is try to watch funny movies to keep my spirits up. It's very hard to be in the consciousness of healing and prayer from that space. This is why I am realizing that I really need extra support and holding, not only on the day of the infusion, but in the more difficult days following it, so I can maintain continuity in my healing and support.

I am open to receive fully and deeply the loving that I deserve and that I am.

I am enormously grateful to all of you for who you are and for the gift of your presence in my life. Please let me know if this is something you feel called to and can be available for, and the times of day that would work best for you.

THANK YOU!

Love,
Tay
XO

Reaching out to my community for help was divinely timed at Imbolc, February 1, a cross-quarter holiday on the Celtic wheel of the year. Imbolc is the time of honoring the goddess Brigid in her maiden form. Brigid is a triple goddess, meaning she represents maiden, mother, and crone aspects of the feminine. Imbolc is the origin of Groundhog Day, the first stirring of springtime. Maiden Brigid carries the flame of healing, connecting us with the younger aspects of ourselves and our innocence and purity within. Feeling divinely inspired to ask for help at this time of year confirmed for me how deeply I am being held and guided by Goddess in this journey. I sensed maiden Brigid lighting a candle in the darkness as I traversed further into the underworld, searching desperately for my own inner maiden, the magical young girl who had been punished and cast away.

MESSAGE TO PRAYER CIRCLE

On a spiritual, soul level, I know this experience is completely about the reclaiming and retrieval of my thirteen-, fourteen-, and fifteen-year-old self. I've learned that it takes cancer approximately twenty years to manifest in the physical body from the time of the original spiritual wound or the loss of soul energy. And for me, that was in my early teenage years.

At that age—most of you know this—I was a sensitive child, very attuned to the mystical and to the energy around me. I began channeling one of my spirit guides on my own, without anyone teaching or guiding me. I was very open and confident about it.

In boarding school, I'd lie down on the floor of the library, open myself up to channel energy, hypnotize my friends, and give them past-life regressions. This came naturally to me; I was simply following my internal impulse. Everything about it felt right. I kept a journal of these youthful sessions, which I still have today. I love to read it occasionally to remind myself of how happy those initial days of discovering my spiritual gifts had been.

However, my blissful, innocent openness and easy willingness to share my gifts with others didn't last long. Some of the students became frightened of me and began to call me a witch, turning my special gifts into something sinister and harmful. I was expelled and put on medication that shut me down for about ten years.

The trauma of this experience, I believe, caused the young mystic I was—who had come into the world flourishing and ready to serve others—to "leave," to go into hiding, even from myself. From my studies and my teachers, I have learned that I experienced a massive loss of my soul energy as a result of this untenable "punishment." A gap was created in my lifeline for the ten-year period I left this part of my young self behind. In this gap, a kind of "antilife energy" existed instead.

This level of trauma is what seeds dis-ease, setting it up to manifest in my body years down the road. There is a powerful opportunity in this for me to get at the root of it all. I'm working on reclaiming that magical, young priestess. This is everything to me.

I've learned through one of the healers and guides I'm working with that I have incarnated with this mission; this is my mission in this life, to reclaim my priestess self from all past lifetimes in which I experienced being shut down from this expression of the truest part of myself.

In this lifetime, I incarnated with a passionate desire to bring my abilities into the world. On a soul level, I was ready to return and express these priestess gifts: the gift of Sight, channeling, and the mystical talents that I was expressing at that tender age. All of these remembered gifts were activated in me with intensity, but I was too young to hold it all. I was too young to contextualize it, or navigate it, or really understand what I was doing.

Then, I went through a rejection similar to so many past lifetimes when I had been exiled, punished, and shamed. When my parents were on the way to pick me up from boarding school, I was afraid they would kill me. Obviously, I was not equipped to understand this kind of profound terror. This level of betrayal and upheaval fragmented my fourteen-year-old self and created the departure of my soul energy that I had been expressing so intensely.

Over the years, to protect myself and get on with my life, I developed a resistance to allowing spiritual energy back in.

At present, I'm working on retrieving that beautiful, powerful, young girl and bringing her back into my world with all of her openness, confidence, clear connection to Spirit, and her ability to bring these gifts in service of healing and for the highest good.

I'm sharing this so that you can help me reach the deepest level of healing available to me. I am asking, from the depth of my heart, for you to help me hold my maiden, my thirteen-, fourteen-, and fifteen-year-old self, with all of her magic, power, and awareness.

Please help me visualize her returning fully and see me retrieving, reintegrating, and reassembling all of the lost soul energy from that time. Because I was without that soul energy from ages fifteen to twenty-five, disconnected from my true self, I am visualizing my lifeline in a linear way. I'm imagining I am pulling all of that soul energy back in and filling in the gaps. The clearest intention you can hold for me is to see me in my complete wholeness.

An affirmation I've been speaking is, "I am liberating myself into wholeness."

As part of this healing, the shedding of my hair was a profound liberation and a release.

It's so strange that I have not missed my hair. Losing it was extremely challenging for me to process; it was terrifying and massive. It took me two months of heavy processing to inwardly prepare for this change to my outward appearance. Now that my hair is gone, it's incredible how okay I've felt. I realize that my hair held a lot of old energy.

My hair is naturally brown, but it was almost gingery brown when I was a kid. For the last ten years or so, I've dyed it lighter. During my magical maiden stage, I dyed it darker. It was almost black at fifteen when I was kicked out of boarding school. But something very intriguing happened during my ceremony to shave my head. Keri, standing there with Ryan, who was so courageously shaving my head, was holding my hair. She said it looked as though it was changing color as it was coming out of my head; it was turning black. I still have the bag of my hair and will send a photo to everyone. The hair in the bag is such a deep, dark brown that it almost looks black; it does not look like the hair that was on my head. Something alchemical and powerful was happening as I shed my locks. The old energy was being pushed out, and she, my young maiden self, was absolutely arriving. I've already had some pretty big experiences of feeling her presence, but there's still a lot of tenderness and vulnerability. I notice when I do feel her trying to express herself, fear appears. I know this is because those memories have been stored with so much fear around them.

I ask for you all to please envision her aligned with me and healed. See us in a sacred, healing space.

Blessed be; thank you all. I love you so very much.

UNCONDITIONAL SUPPORT

Every day this group of women—living examples of unconditional love, support, and true sisterhood—lifted me up. After our daily meditations, our What's App group chat would flood with messages describing the beautiful visuals and powerful sensations that each had experienced. Some friends left me messages weeping with gratitude and thanking me for the opportunity to participate in such a magnificent energy field. I was consistently blown away! At different times, each woman shared with me how meaningful it was to experience the palpable energy of pure support. We were all deeply moved by the healing container we were cocreating.

"Tay, last night's meditation was profound. I closed my eyes, and I was in the circle. You were in the center, and we were all chanting and dancing and doing ancient witchy movements around you. Streams of light were twirling around and through you, and through each sister. I am blown away at the potency. Can't wait to circle in an hour. Loving you, seeing you in your vitality, standing with you in your vibrant health and well-being." ~ Maura

"The rituals that are transpiring in this space are truly magical, dear Sister! I cherish these gatherings and look forward to each one." ~ Gigi

"Wow, wow, wow, wow, wow! Thank you so much for calling on us! Thank you for sharing your journey and all of the sacred details! Thank you for being YOU! No words to really acknowledge the profundity of the work that is taking place. Deeply honored to be one of the women called to be present for you. Love you!" ~ Ashley

MESSAGE TO PRAYER CIRCLE

I am crying reading your beautiful visions! Feeling all of it so potently. I experienced being bathed in golden/white/silvery light, my light body expansive and strong, and all cancer cells completely disappearing. I also felt a dragon within me working with the medicine to support me in the transformation. Brigid's presence was there, so strong and powerful, embracing us all as her daughters. So grateful. Love you all so very much.

My dear friends in prayer circle walked with me every step of the way, supporting me through all the phases of understanding. In the beginning, my mission was to avoid surgery, imagining healing miracles occurring during chemo. Together, we meditated on an image of a healthy mammogram with healthy breast tissue. We got so detailed that we created a specific scenario for my midtreatment check-in with Dr. Funk. After three of six rounds of chemo, I went in for an ultrasound to check the progress. My oncologist had encouraged me not to get my hopes up, as usually nothing changes from the picture this quickly, yet that doesn't mean the treatment isn't working. He said sometimes dead cells take up the same amount of mass as the tumor. My prayer circle and I vividly imagined a clear ultrasound and Dr. Funk exclaiming, "There's no cancer!"

When I went in for this appointment, after pressing the ultrasound wand to my chest, she said, "Wow, you are responding so well to this therapy," and after a moment exclaimed, "Seriously, Taylor, what cancer?"

It was like living through a dream. I immediately wrote to my prayer circle and could practically hear the hooting and hollering vibrating through their responses as they arrived on my phone.

MESSAGE TO PRAYER CIRCLE, AS I WAS LEAVING THE DOCTOR

Some really good news, sisters! I'm seriously amazed and in awe of the power of this prayer circle! There is no visible cancer in my nodes or in the spot in my breast that was first biopsied! They put a clip in it during the biopsy and all that was visible on the ultrasound today was the clip—otherwise healthy tissue! My doctor said, "Seriously, Taylor, what cancer? There's nothing here!" She also gave me another biopsy on a different spot on my breast that had been visible previously on the mammogram image but hadn't been biopsied—major prayers needed for those results.

The last part of my message described the unexpected part of my visit with Dr. Funk—that she had decided to do one more biopsy of a spot that had been seen on the original mammogram image but not yet biopsied. She phoned me the next evening to share the results: it was also invasive cancer. Another tumor. At first, this took the wind out of my sails.

MESSAGES FROM PRAYER CIRCLE, IN RESPONSE TO THE NEWLY DISCOVERED TUMOR

"Deeply feeling you, sister. I hear how hard this feels right now. But your way is still clearing. Two steps forward, one step back. You are still moving forward. Love you so much, Lady of the Lake." ~ Keri

"Holding you, dear sister Tay, in your fierce grace and loving intention for healing and miracles on all levels. Also calling in healing for Dr. Funk and Dr. Piro so they may be in divine alignment with the miracle that you are! Big miracles are coming! I feel it! I'm in awe of the light your soul is calling in for you and all of us. Thank you for your courage and strength and your beautiful heart. You inspire and heal me daily on many levels. Big love to your blessed breasts and body. I love you, sister. This healing circle itself is a miracle of love and light. I'm overwhelmed with gratitude for you, sisters. Truly." ~ Val

"This morning I'm imagining you being filled with golden yellow light. This light is clarifying your body's intention and determination in dissolving any mass invading your body, mind, and heart. Golden wings of light and love emerge and hold you. You are held. You are loved. You are forever pure and true." ~ Ashni

"Holding you in so much fierce love and tender care." ~ Harmony

"Oh, Tay, I acknowledge the painful intrusions on your beautiful body and the disappointments you are feeling right now, and I deeply honor your bravery in holding these experiences along with the miracles and light being poured in and around you. What an expansive container you have created to be able to hold this all. Thank you for your honesty and tenderness, Tay. We are standing with you as a reflection of your strength while you navigate all that is unfolding and as you continue moving toward more healing, more growth, and more expansion. You are so, so loved and held." ~ Caroline

One of my sisters responded that we simply did not know this third tumor was there, so we hadn't known to focus our healing energy on it. Everyone agreed that now that it had been brought to our attention, it was time to do our work! Look how well the other two had responded. This attitude brought me relief. I imagined a rake combing the bottom of the sea, unearthing artifacts from times past and watching them float up to the surface. The healing energy being showered through me was moving through the layers of my consciousness like this rake in the bottom of the sea, unearthing what needed to be seen and remembered for me to align with the purity of my being.

The next time I went for a chemo infusion, accompanied by my dear friend, April, my prayer circle sister, Baelyn, sent the following message:

> *"Taylor, I was reflecting on this quote from Starhawk as I was listening to you speak and communicate, and appreciating your power and clarity with your words: 'Language shapes consciousness and the use of language to shape consciousness is an important branch of magic.' So, I was thinking...maybe you can create a mantra or short affirmation that is of the highest vibration to you, and we can all have that to invoke and chant for you aloud from wherever we are, whether in moments of prayer circle or anytime throughout the day, throughout your treatment, and at any point in this journey. If this resonates, I would love to know your mantra and sing it loud, speak it out, hold it in my heart, and sing it softly to you as the journey weaves and continues to unfold. Maybe we can all do the same?"* ~ Baelyn

Sitting with April in the hospital room with chemo flowing through my veins, I thought about my affirmations and healing intentions. I was becoming more aware of a strong divine feminine presence guiding me, whispering to me in my dreams and meditations. She described herself this way:

I am multidimensional. I am personal while also being an archetypal energy. In Avalon, many women have reigned as the Lady of the Lake. All are similar to a reigning queen on a throne. An energy imbues each woman as a whole, and yet each woman holds significant wisdom and memories relevant to her particular time as the Lady of the Lake.

What would become my healing song came through in a burst of inspiration and April sent the following message to our healing circle:

"Hi, magic team! We can both feel you here; it's incredible to experience this love from all of you! Tay's intention is to release all dimensions and densities that do not serve her divinity. Here is her mantra:

I am in absolute devotion

To my divinity

I am the living spirit within

I am the living embodiment

of the Goddess

I am the Lady of the Lake

Lady of the Lake, rise

Lady of the Lake, rise

Lady of the Lake, rise!*

"Love, love, love you! Feeling us circled around you, softly chanting your mantra to you all day as this radiant healing light enters your body and swirls through you, transforming your cells into their highest expression of wellness with a vortex of energy sending the unhealthy cells down into Mother Earth and up into Father Sky." ~ Gigi

LIVING BETWEEN THE WORLDS

As I progressed further into treatment, I experienced the cumulative effect of chemo taking its toll. Right before my third round, after I had completed three out of six infusions, I had an especially powerful session with Chung Fu. He guided me on a vision journey to a healing temple on Avalon, where I was escorted to a room in which spirit doctors were preparing for surgery. A group of nurses who felt like ancient priestesses and medicine women prepared me, bathing me, changing me into a white gown, burning incense, and rubbing herbal ointments over my skin. The spirit doctors performed a psychic surgery, operating on me etherically and removing remnants of the three tumors from my body. Although this took place in the inner planes, I felt pressure in my physical body and experienced soreness for a few days after. This psychic surgery was a success, and when we were complete, Chung Fu guided me to a place I had been before, that we both referred to as my spirit garden. My spirit garden was a sanctuary where I could go at any time to experience peace. I saw altars dedicated to the elements, adorned with feathers and incense smoke for air, candle flames honoring fire, amethyst crystals for earth, and a chalice overflowing with sacred water. The healing tones of crystal singing bowls resonated throughout the sanctuary and the air smelled of rose and frankincense. As I stood in my spirit garden, I realized I was my fifteen-year-old self. I felt strong, empowered, resilient, and healthy.

A long silver cape was draped over my body, a sword raised in the air from my outstretched right arm, a shield protecting my left chest. The power of the earth surged through my bare feet, and I gazed around to see flowers bursting in a circle around me in every color of the rainbow. When I returned from this journey and our session completed, I sat on the floor with colored pencils and drew the image of my silver-caped maiden with flowers of every color of the rainbow around her, from red to purple. I called her my rainbow warrior priestess.

A few days later, as I was recovering from my third round of chemo, flowers were delivered to my home: a bouquet of red flowers from my prayer circle sisters. The next day, another arrangement was delivered; this time the flowers were orange. On the third day, a yellow arrangement arrived. On the fourth day, the bouquet was green. Day after day this continued as I received gorgeous blooms of blue, purple, and white, each bouquet sent from prayer circle sisters. The images from the inner planes were appearing in the outer world! I had not shared my experience with the rainbow warrior priestess with anyone. The experience of receiving something in physical world reality that so exactly echoed the healing images of my inner world was a powerful confirmation from the spirit realms of the truth of the healing that was occurring. The veil had been lifted, and I was coexisting in different worlds.

MESSAGES FROM SISTERS, THE WEEK THE FLOWERS WERE ARRIVING

"Oh, Tay! Those orange blooms sound divine. I was watching my goddaughter tonight, and when reading her a story, out of nowhere she started saying, 'Flower power!' I've never heard her say that before. Beaming you love and prayers for abundant, limitless grace in the days ahead. I hope the kitties are snuggled up right next to you! Love you, and love you all." ~ Bonne

"I am so happy you're basking in the love that is radiating from those flowers! We love you." ~ Jenny

"Loving you so much, goddess! We are with you! Singing to your heart through the energy of the flowers surrounding you!" ~ Ashley

As treatments became more intense, my friend Harmony created a schedule for sisters to come sit with me so I wouldn't have to try to organize visitors, and someone would always be available during a specific time each day. This provided such invaluable support. For an hour or two, one of my friends would sit by my side, sometimes in silence as I slept, or rubbing my feet, or telling me stories about things happening in the outside world.

"Knowing what is happening locally to support Tay helps me hold the vision for us all. Radiating love to Tay, all the healing circle sisters, and Taylor's whole support team. Loving you, Tay." ~ Ange

WISDOM

Biopsy

I'm on my back on the medical table, my gown open at the front. My breasts are exposed. My doctor leans over me with a large biopsy needle and injects it deep into the skin above my left nipple. It feels like being punched with a staple gun. The pressure on my breastplate is so immense at first that it is as though the wind is being knocked out of me.

As I walk through the fourth gate of the underworld, I am being stripped of the breastplate from my heart. Protective tendencies that had prevented me from fully exposing the rawness of my emotions are dismantled. I am wide open, seen, revealing my wounds, grief, sadness, and the shadows I have kept hidden within my heart. To truly give and receive love, the misunderstanding that I could do it all on my own or keep things inside with no consequence must melt away in the bubbling cauldron I am swimming in. I am learning the powerful lesson of asking for what I need and learning to receive and accept it. I am learning that I am worthy of receiving the love that I am being given. I am learning to listen to my own truthful needs instead of always trying to make it comfortable for everyone else. I am beginning to listen to myself and discover what my needs are—needs that have been hidden underneath the protective breast-plate of the person who never wanted to displease anyone.

INANNA'S DESCENT

Gate 4: Removal of the Breastplate: Withholding Love

As Inanna approaches the fourth gate of the underworld, having been stripped of her crown, her lapis lazuli, and the double strand of beads around her neck, she is now adorned only from her chest down. The gatekeeper demands that her breastplate be removed. The breastplate sheltered the vulnerable energy center of her heart chakra, located at the center of her chest. Inanna asks, "What is this?" Once more, she is told: "Quiet, Inanna; the ways of the under-world are perfect. They may not be questioned."

Inanna is stripped of the protection around her heart, from the familiarity of giving and receiving love according to the conditions of the upperworld, the place where she felt comfortable and in con-trol. In the underworld, the rules of the upperworld do not apply, and the wild and unknown places of her heart are exposed.

Journal Entry from the Lady of the Lake to Me

Merge with me in my deep, crystal-clear healing waters that are mir-rors of your reflection. See yourself as a pure being of radiant light, wisdom, majesty, and truth with all impurities dissolved. See us as one integrated being.

You are one of the Ladies of the Lake; your soul has sat with me over many lifetimes. As you go deeper into this exploration, you shall tap into my wisdom and also receive help from beings on the other side, as well as in Avalon. This is destined to come through you, beloved. This is what you have come here to do. You are ready. The time has come. Blessed be.

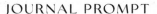

JOURNAL PROMPT

Do you allow yourself to receive? Compliments, gifts, loving, affection?

As a child, how did your family express their loving? Have you inherited this way of being? Do you feel you openly share the love in your heart? Are you in touch with that?

MEDITATION

Sit comfortably with your spine straight, or lie down, where you will not be disturbed.

Close your eyes, and begin taking in deep diaphragmatic breaths, in through the nose, filling and expanding the belly, and out through the mouth with an audible exhale...ahhh. Repeat three times.

Bring your hands to the center of your chest, your heart center.

Your heart center governs the acts of giving and receiving love. It is a place of profound wisdom, a treasure trove of your deepest truths.

Ask your heart to reveal to you what has been in the way of your giving and receiving love unconditionally. What fears, conditioning, or limiting beliefs are held there? What messages have you given yourself about receiving love? Do you feel unworthy?

At what age did your heart close to its full expression?

Allow yourself to receive any memories or impressions that arise, and trust them. Do not analyze or overthink this. What age is present?

Visualize this younger version of yourself standing alongside Inanna, at the fourth gate of the underworld. You notice this younger aspect of you is wearing a breastplate over their heart, just as Inanna was. To reveal the treasure chest that was buried beneath this protective covering, the breastplate must be released into the underworld. As your younger self and Inanna cross this threshold, the breastplate dissolves. Through opening to give and receive love fully, the key to the treasure will be uncovered.

Bring your awareness back to your hands at your heart center. Visualize a beautiful green energy expanding out from this space, with soft pink and rainbow hues sparkling in its sphere.

Set the intention to open to give and receive greater levels of love in your life.

Take a deep breath, sowing the seed of this intention into your heart space.

When you are ready, open your eyes and journal any insights that came forward.

Blessed be.

Chapter Five

LIGHT INFUSION

FIFTH GATE: POWER

"Life shrinks or expands in proportion to one's courage."

~ Anaïs Nin

MESSAGE TO FRIENDS AND FAMILY, THE DAY AFTER FIRST CHEMO TREATMENT

Before having cancer, I thought of chemo as poison, and the little I knew of it sounded horrendous. The only way I could accept this substance into my body and let it do the work that needed to be done was to change the way I related to it. I decided to reframe the chemo as sacred medicine, and Alisha helped me come up with the term "light infusion," which brought forward a comforting feeling.

Yesterday, I received my first round of chemo, or light infusion. I was blessed to have my close friend Val by my side throughout the incredibly long day. Three of my dearest soul sisters have come together to create a "chemo support plan" and are taking turns being with me during these light infusions, holding a nurturing and sacred space for the deepest level of healing to occur. I received neck and foot massages, had stories from Clarissa Pinkola Estés's Women Who Run with the Wolves read aloud to me, and was guided through healing visualizations and prayers. I am so grateful for this support and know it's already helping me profoundly. As strange as this may sound, I actually felt inspired and nourished during the light infusion yesterday! Inspired by the power of love. Val held my hand, without making anything wrong or bad, or pitying me. She simply sat beside me, her presence reminding me of my truth and power. I am a divine being having a human experience. I am not a victim. I am here to learn and grow spiritually and for whatever reason, this dis-ease is part of the curriculum I have chosen. I was nourished by the palpable support I experienced as loving text messages flooded in from friends and family. The energy of support and love I felt expanded beyond the walls of the hospital, beyond the pain and fear of the physical circumstances and environment. It made me understand from the inside out that anything can be made into a beautiful experience if we change the way we relate to it.

. . .

I imagined angels administering a high vibration liquid light medicine that flowed gracefully through my body, clearing karma, healing wounds, and releasing toxic emotions or negativity along with all trace of dis-ease from any level of my consciousness. To support this intention, Alisha suggested I focus on healing images while I was receiving the treatments, images that would take me to a place of comfort and peace inside. Whenever I was afraid or anxious, I placed my hands on my body, one hand on my belly and one on my heart, and called on Blue's soul to be with me. As I sat receiving my first light infusion, I closed my eyes and flashed from one image to the next:

Blue and my childhood pony, Misty, together in an expansive green pasture, with my inner child.

Standing under St. Nectan's Glen, an enchanting waterfall in Tintagel, Cornwall, feeling the water rush through me, turning into golden light.

Bathing in the water of the Chalice Well, standing naked with my arms outstretched, looking up into the branches of the trees and breathing in the cool, crisp air, embraced by the love of the land of Avalon.

The first day was a very long day that began with an echocardiogram, something I would receive every three months for one year to make sure my heart was tolerating the medication well. Before my blood was drawn and the IV inserted, the nurse read all the potential frightening side effects of each of the four medicines I would be receiving. Imagine the end of a pharmaceutical commercial rattling on for thirty minutes. I continued to hold my body and see my healing images, calling on Blue's soul to be with me for comfort and strength.

Because it was the first round and they didn't know how I would respond, they administered a dose of Benadryl so high that it felt like I had ingested psychedelic plant medicine. I closed my eyes and saw myself in the Hermitage Hall, an area of my dorm in ninth grade that was surrounded in rumors and urban-legend ghost stories. Kids whispered of a student who had hung himself in one of the two rooms down this tiny hallway that was so small in comparison to all the other dorms and buildings on the campus. The Hermitage Hall was off the beaten track, away from the comfort of all the other rooms in my girls' dorm, yet everyone knew this ghost story.

When I was in ninth grade, kids made up rumors about me—that I would stay up late at night casting spells and practicing magic in the Hermitage Hall. In truth, I was as spooked by this hallway as all the others. I hadn't thought about this place for over twenty years, yet as my body received her first dose of these potent medicines, I closed my eyes and was engulfed by an experience of being there. I was in the Hermitage Hall, and Blue was with me. We were going to retrieve my fourteen-year-old self. I kicked open the door and there she was, tied up in the scary room, bound and gagged, with an apple in her mouth. It was time to completely retrieve her. I cut the ropes from her hands and feet and released the gag from her mouth, and together we jumped up onto Blue's back and rode away. *I am here to save you! To rescue you from the shadows and rumors and misunderstandings. I'm sorry I left you for so long. I hear you now! I have come!* I realized the power of other people's words and the effect those rumors had on me at that tender and vulnerable age. They banished part of me to that hall, where an aspect of my young self who had been traumatized at this school had remained stunted.

Val sat on a small chair next to me during this long first day at the hospital. We were in a crowded room with others also receiving chemo. Her comforting and protective presence shielded me, surrounding us in a bubble of light throughout the day. As I lay in the chair with the IV in my arm and the freezing cold ice cap on my head, drool falling from my lips as I dozed in and out of awareness, she lovingly swiped her fingers across my face, reminding me I was wearing my warrior paint.

After this first experience, I asked for a private room and was so thankful to receive it. One of my three beloved sisters from my light infusion team would come with me, and we would wipe down all the surfaces, lay an altar cloth over the table, and decorate the room with crystals and sacred objects. We brought flowers, aromatherapy, and scarves to hang over the computer screens. We turned off the fluorescent light and let the natural light shine in from the window. We said prayers inviting Goddess, my guides, and angels to charge the room with love and healing energy. Every time a nurse walked in, she would pause, taking in the space, often commenting on its beauty or how good it smelled.

When they brought in bags of medicine, I asked if I could please hold the medicine bag before they administered it. I wanted to tune the medicine to my body and ask that my body receive it with grace, ease, and healing. My light infusion friend and I held our hands over the bags together, wearing gloves because the potency is that strong, even inside an IV bag. We sent our love and prayers into these bags. I held each bag to my body, visualizing it as sacred medicine my body needed to cleanse and clear karma, and purge negativity, imbalance, and any trace of dis-ease from me. I also envisioned a shungite shield, a powerful black stone used for protection, around all my organs. I asked the medicine to be directed specifically to where it needed to go, not harming anything else.

OPENING TO CHANNEL

From the beginning, Alisha saw the importance of me opening to my channeling abilities again, and we began exercises to help me with this right away. At first, she asked me to receive messages and speak them aloud during our sessions. In our first session, she had me close my eyes, clear my mind, and ask Goddess, *How do I transform treatment into a spiritual opportunity?* This is what came through me:

> *My child, release the misunderstanding that you've done something wrong. This path will lead you to beautiful places. See the medicine absolving the misunderstanding that you can't get it right, absolving all limiting beliefs and misunderstandings from your heart. See the word "wrong" being pushed out of your body and consciousness by the light of this medicine.*

I loved the image of the word "wrong" leaving my body completely. During light infusion treatments, as I placed my gloved hands over the IV bag, I imagined black-and-white words like newspaper print with the word "wrong" written on it being purged from my body, mind, and spirit.

Alisha and I worked with my inner fourteen-year-old every week. In my vision, I would go to her dorm room and talk with her there, until eventually, the environment changed. First it was a stark hospital-like room, then more of a nice hotel with a beautiful bath-room, and then her healing sanctuary where she lay on sheepskins in front of a cozy fire. In the beginning, I would see my young self in a deep sleep. Then, I remember the day she first stirred. It aligned with the season of Imbolc, celebrating the maiden Brigid and mark-ing the first stirring of spring, when the light begins to increase after the long dark days of winter. The maiden Brigid is an awakener who ignites the flame of inspiration and stands at the threshold of new beginnings. During my quiet Imbolc ceremony outside the tree house that held us during my treatment, Brigid came to me:

Bring your inner maiden to me. Bring her to my mantel of healing. Allow me to cleanse her in my sacred waters and purify her in my forge. I will help you heal this precious and sacred aspect of yourself, my daughter, my sweet daughter. You are safe, forever in my embrace. There is nothing to be feared. Come to me. Lay your worries at my feet.

I felt my magical maiden within awaken from her long slumber during this time. After she stirred, she was angry, and I sat with her as she screamed and shouted at me for ignoring her for so long. I promised I was here now for good, that she had my full attention, and that I was willing to do whatever it took to allow her full expres-sion within me. She showered and cleansed herself, dressed in vio-let and silver robes, and settled into the sacred space of her healing sanctuary.

. . .

I hadn't realized that up until that point, I had lived my adult life with a gaping absence of my soul energy, a loss of power, truth, and presence, that I had been severed from a truth so pure and real within that I had never been freely, authentically me. I hadn't even known that I was disempowered, that my power had been stripped from me twenty-one years ago, and lifetimes before that. The power of the light infusion was showing me where my power had *not* been;

the loss of safety and freedom in my spiritual expression showed me where I had been vacant, empty. Seeing it this way allowed me to understand why I made the choices I did in my late teens and early twenties, when my body was filled with medications and recreational drugs, and my spirit energy was not fully there to guide me. I marveled at the miracle of getting this far, of knowing there was something that needed to be reclaimed, without knowing precisely what that thing was. Sitting with a needle in my arm and a hospital bracelet around my wrist, I knew that cancer had not disempowered me. I had been stripped of my power long before the cancer arrived.

INANNA'S DESCENT

Gate 5: Loss of the Gold Bracelet: Power

As Inanna enters the fifth gate of the underworld, the gold bracelet from her wrist is removed. Once more she is told, "Quiet, Inanna; the ways of the underworld are perfect. They may not be questioned."

The fifth gate is connected to the solar plexus, the energy center that is the seat of the emotions, personal power, will, and identity. Inanna's gold bracelet represents her power in the upper world, her command over her queendom. The underworld cracks open the shadow gate of her solar plexus, revealing unseen and well-hidden emotional trauma, disempowerment, and disowned aspects of her consciousness.

As Inanna walks further into the underworld, she experiences a great sense of loss of something more profound than her gold bracelet, of something she hadn't even known she was missing. Neither of us knew that an aspect of ourselves had been lost until our attention was drawn to the place of the wound. My gold bracelet was removed in my teen years, yet I was not able to access the memory until the hospital bracelet was there to replace it. Inanna's gold bracelet represented her power and authority over her domain in the upper world, yet as it was taken away, she was filled with memories of a deeper, truer source of power that comes from inside her.

MEDITATION EXPERIENCE

In my meditation today, I journeyed into the Avalonian temple of me, where my fourteen-year-old dwells in her robes. She was lounging with the souls/higher selves of Mom; Dad; my sister, Sheila; and my brother, Wells. There was a beautiful spiral staircase that led me down to a room glowing with moonstone and morganite light. I heard a ritual outside and walked to hear priestesses chanting in the night in a ceremony and singing, "The earth, the air, the fire, the water, return, return, return, return..." and the chorus went on, "Return, return, return, return, return, return, return."

I asked what the ceremony was for and my young self said, "It's for you. They are preparing you for your return." I saw myself as the Lady of the Lake lying on a beautiful wooden bed, a pyre, surrounded in flowers, herbs, and incense, and they were singing and chanting around me. Then, I walked out and saw Avalon, gloriously beautiful majestic mountains of emerald green and a stone circle in the valley to the right. Women were dancing and twirling in sync in a ritual. Birds flew overhead and misty clouds moved between the mountains of lush green.

JOURNALING

Alisha encouraged me to start a daily journal where I began by writing a minute or two of self-forgiveness—whatever was present in that moment—and afterward, channeling a message from my higher Self—my heart, my breast, whatever I felt drawn to. The more I kept my journal, the deeper I seemed to go, trusting the area of my body that was asking to be given a voice. Twice a day, as I sat at my altar after prayer circle, I wrote in my journal. At first, messages from my body came forward, ones that contained great wisdom. But soon, an opening was created for messages from the Lady of the Lake, as well.

JOURNAL ENTRY

I forgive myself for buying into the misunderstanding that I am wrong.

I forgive myself for all judgments associated with being wrong, bad, stupid.

I forgive myself for judging myself as wrong for channeling, as wrong for anything I've done in the past.

I forgive and release all judgments against myself as wrong.

MESSAGE FROM MY HEART

The divine intelligence that I am is "beyond right-doing or wrongdoing," my sweet angel. The eternal love that pours forth from the source that feeds me is never ending. I am attuned with and connected to the frequency of divine love straight from the heart of Goddess. All hearts truly do beat as one in this sense. We are all emanations and transmitters of the supreme love from Source. The human experience gets in the way of the transmission of this Love.

I forgive myself for judging myself as self-righteous.

I forgive myself for judging myself as putting myself in danger.

I forgive myself for judging myself as doing something wrong.

I forgive myself for judging myself as doing something wrong or bad and not being able to trust my inner guidance.

I forgive myself for judging myself and buying into all judgments associated with not being able to trust my inner guidance.

MESSAGE FROM MY CROWN

I am opening to receive higher frequencies of divine light, wisdom, and information. I am being recalibrated following the shedding of my hair. The opening has created a powerful opportunity to reactivate centers in my body and soul consciousness that have been closed for a very long time—beyond this lifetime. Allow this process to unfold. It is done in perfect timing.

I forgive and release the guilt and grief in my heart around my beloved Blue.

I forgive all judgments against myself of not being a good enough mom, caretaker, provider, of not being enough.

I forgive myself for constantly feeling I wasn't doing enough.

I let go of all the guilt in my heart.

I forgive myself for all judgments against my mothering of Blue, and release and forgive all parts of myself that hold guilt and grief.

I forgive myself fully and completely, and feel the release from my heart in this moment.

MESSAGE FROM MY THIRD EYE

I am open. My gift of Sight has been restored and I rejoice. I rejoice in this miracle and reconciliation of a karmic wound. A powerful and profound healing has occurred. I am stirring awake, reactivating and calibrating, and you will soon remember how to access me. All will come forward into your awareness and waking consciousness soon. You are being restored. You are here! A sacred day to be certain. Blessed be.

I forgive myself for judging my maiden self as destructive or self-righteous.

I forgive all energies connected to that line of energy from other lifetimes.

I forgive myself for judging myself as not seeing my maiden's innocence.

I forgive myself for judging the purity of her connection and transmission.

MESSAGE FROM MY LEFT BREAST

I love you. I am acting in service of your highest destiny and soul's potential in this lifetime. I am calling you to higher levels of awakening and experience. I am uniting all lost or disassembled aspects of your spirit. I am here in service to your soul's mission, your divine plan. I am not here to hurt you, and I have no agenda around staying. I see you doing your work. I am transmuting the unhealthy cells as you work.

After these messages from my body, I began to communicate clearly with the Lady of the Lake *and* the Lady of Avalon. In my experience, the Lady of the Lake embodies the collective consciousness of all priestess teachers who once served on the Isle of Avalon, keeping the mysteries and passing them down. My soul has served this role, and I am part of that collective. The Lady of the Lake, and those memories, are awakening within me and bringing forward my ancient priestess self. The Lady of Avalon is the goddess of the Isle of Avalon, whose spirit dwells there in the landscape.

JOURNAL ENTRY

Lady of the Lake: *It's not about being "special." It's about being real and true to who you are and what you're here to bring through.*

SESSION WITH CHUNG FU

I worked with Alisha every week and Chung Fu over the phone once every three weeks, which was the length between rounds of chemo.

Chung Fu: Continue with the work you've been doing, in which you see your chemo as light, as a golden substance being welcomed into your body, coming in and flowing into the two remaining spots of cancer. Be quite specific about this in your vision. Do this at least two or three times a week and really get inside your breast. Draw the chemo into those two places, especially on the actual day the chemo is coming in. Envision this as though you're inside your breast, like a traffic cop—"no, this way, over here, turn left, in there"—as though you can literally guide the stream of it to those two areas. It's also very good for you to get practice using your muscles of visualization when you have something very specific to work with, as you do now.

Directing the chemo in this way will help you manage it on the inside of your body. When you try and turn away from it—I don't think you have at all, but some people do—it gets harder; when you try to pretend it's not happening, or refuse it, or push it back, it gets harder. This type of drug has a terrific force and can block your energy, so it's good to practice directing it to the areas it can be usefully employed instead of allowing it to roam freely in your body.

I was happy to receive this concrete visualization about directing the chemo and knew I could follow through with his suggestions.

Going to see the doctor is always quite a big thing, isn't it? You have to sit with "the man who knows." The medically trained man who is going to tell you things, give you information about your body, your light infusion, your breast, and tell you how you are doing in the middle of your treatment. This brings up many complicated feelings.

I nodded my head yes. He was so right about the anxiety the doctor visits brought up. Even though my doctors were compassionate, it was extremely challenging to stay centered while hearing results. In such a traumatized state, it was easy to give my power away to their words and become very emotional, even though my intention was to stay strong and trust in the knowing that I would heal completely.

You've been through a lot, and it's not over. Although the doctors and people in authority are taking care of you, it's actually pretty painful to go through. This is not a joyride—managing the feelings it brings up is quite a lot. This is a bit reminiscent of your teen years when your parents thought they were taking care of you while allowing you to take powerful drugs that affected your psyche and shut you down. Chung Fu wishes there were less aggressive drugs available in your world, but at the moment, there aren't. This treatment that can be brutal will change over time.

I was grateful that Chung Fu acknowledged the power of chemo, reminding me that I was passing through a physically and emotionally grueling medical regimen that would be hard for anyone. I needed to be very gentle with myself.

You came into your life not really knowing about empowerment and connection to Source. It's as though you've just been shaken along, bumping along the track. This illness and your adolescent betrayal have tested your faith all the way. And I think your faith is very strong, dear one.

I knew he was right and this felt good. "When you speak about the connection to my younger self, I feel it in my bones so deeply. Something has shifted and the floodgates have opened, allowing me to be able to make those connections and access those feelings."

Well done. This is happening for you through a combination of the support and encouragement you have now. And you're making the connection with Goddess. You have my voice, but you also have your own connection working on the inside. Now, you are joining your priestess, witch, and magical shamanka places. You're bringing your wounded child into this higher level of self-expression. This is giving her hope. The hopelessness that has resided inside for so long is the reason you've wanted to do this "big healing." You asked for healing—don't forget— way before you knew you had cancer. That's right. You're getting more and more in touch with yourself, going inside and finding these places that need healing. Your sense of empowerment will continue to burst through after the treatment. It will happen authentically, with Goddess. I can see this happening. This is wonderful, dear one.

"I am so grateful to hear you say this," I replied. "Knowing that these healings and awakenings will burst through in a conscious way after the fog of the chemo has lifted gives me a glimmer of excitement and hope."

JOURNAL ENTRY

I dreamed last night that Jane Fonda was giving me an award for courage and bravery, a warrior award for women who are inspirations and examples to others. I woke up and cried as I told Ryan about it. I was holding a tissue up to my bloody nose as I cried. I do deserve an award! In the dream, I felt inspired to start an organization for warrior goddesses and give out similar awards to acknowledge strong women.

JOURNAL PROMPT

Where in your life do you feel you hold power? Is it through your job, family, finances, talents, relationships, or something else? What if that were taken away?

MEDITATION

Sit comfortably with your spine straight, or lie down, where you will not be disturbed.

Close your eyes, and begin taking in deep diaphragmatic breaths, in through the nose, filling and expanding the belly, and out through the mouth with an audible exhale...ahhh. Repeat three times.

Place your hands at your solar plexus, the chakra that rests at the center of your rib cage, a few inches above your belly button. This center vibrates to a golden yellow frequency that is warm like the sun. Visualize the sun shining beneath your hands and a warm feeling being generated from there.

This center is the seat of your power, emotions, and relationship with yourself.

When in your life do you place judgments against yourself? Do you ever judge yourself as weak, bad, or wrong?

Experience those judgments rumbling up to the surface and erupting like lava rocks from a volcano. These rocks have been filling a void within you, hiding away something you hadn't been in touch with before. What is underneath those judgments?

See Inanna standing before you with a large bucket. She is collecting these rocks as they spill over onto the floor in front of you. As the bucket is filling up, you become aware of an absence within this energy center. Where does it lead? What has it revealed? Trust whatever feelings or impressions arise.

When the bucket is filled to the brim with these black lava rocks, Inanna carries it over the threshold of the fifth gate of the underworld. This release enables you to remember what these rocks had been carefully hiding, preserving something within you in a wounded state; the parts of you that were banished as wrong, bad, or unworthy.

Take some time to lovingly send compassionate self-forgiveness into your solar plexus now.

To your surprise, something beautiful appears, a healing image full of strength and courage. Receive this impression and allow it to wash over you, cleansing any residue from the black rocks that were released.

Come back to your breath and trust that the power of the underworld will support you in retrieving what had been previously hidden or lost.

When you are ready, open your eyes, and on a blank page, write down any of the false beliefs or judgments that came forward. Once they are down on the page, tear up the paper or burn it in a fireplace, without reading it a second time. This will assist the transmutation of the energy that has been released. Repeat this practice as often as you wish.

Blessed be.

Chapter Six

SHADOWS OF THE SPIRITUAL COMMUNITY

SIXTH GATE: GIVING OTHERS SPIRITUAL AUTHORITY

"The biggest authority on you is always you."

~ Alisha Das Hayes

GIVING UP MY SOVEREIGNTY

I experienced cancer as a truth serum. It showed me the energetic dynamics that had been unconsciously playing out in my life for years, with the recurring theme that I had given my power away. This new awareness elevated certain feelings that had been tucked away just below my conscious thought—hunches I had about people or situations—and spelled them out for me, as if displayed on a neon sign right in front of my face. This potent "truth medicine" resulted in the dismantling of relationships with people I had related to as spiritual authority figures, tearing down the illusion that another person could ever know what's best for me.

Unknowingly, I had placed my power and authority in the hands of others, relying on guidance and advice from those whom I perceived to be more clearly connected to Spirit than I was. I was not consciously aware of this pattern at the time because I was coming from a place of self-doubt and unworthiness. My desire to strengthen myself spiritually was pure, but I had not yet cultivated trust in myself. Emotionally, I was vulnerable and raw, in the beginning stages of peeling the layers of bandages from neglected, festering wounds. I was seeking teachers, support and guidance from those who had walked the path before me. This became deeply confusing because I *did* receive significant healing support from these figures. However, sometimes the guidance I heard went against my own intuition, or the feelings in my heart. I often experienced inner conflict and anxiety when I felt my behavior or choices were met with disapproval, and many times, this led me to choose against what was true in my own heart. I struggled with this cycle of inner turmoil for years.

SPIRITUAL TEACHERS

Nicholas

I met Nicholas, an exorcist in his seventies, at a time in my life when I was desperate to clear the energies of my past experiences and start fresh. My early twenties were spent entrenched in the shadows of drugs and alcohol. I had painfully low self-esteem and was constantly seeking experiences to feel connected and validated. The Ritalin use in my teens progressed to Adderall, which eventually led to cocaine. The benefit I received from being high was the temporary numbing of all the pain and separation I felt inside. And, for a few hours, with the right friends, I could talk about spirituality freely. I remember sitting in bed with my best friend and roommate, Molly, and her saying to me, "Tay, I think you're a healer. Even in such darkness, you carry so much light. I can't imagine what you would be like without all this darkness."

Thankfully, Molly, along with two other friends, my aunt, and my mom, arranged an intervention just after my twenty-fourth birthday. My time in treatment immediately opened me to the possibility of connecting with the magical young teen I had been. I remember writing in my journal about how my angels had guided me to that facility, and I was so grateful my friends had done for me something I didn't know how to do for myself. I know that through the deep emotional work combined with the energetic clearing and healing I experienced in the years that followed, I expelled toxic residue from my consciousness and transcended addiction.

Around the time I met Nicholas, at age twenty-six, I was actively seeking pathways to healing. Nicholas's realm of mastery was energetic extractions, also known as exorcisms. I had not sought out an exorcist; I met Nicholas through another healer I had a few sessions with, who directed me to him. Nicholas is very unconventional in his methods and as he works, he makes sounds that can be quite frightening. He says it's the energy passing through him, and the first time I worked with him in person, I saw that was true. He would morph and shape-shift as he worked, and while he cleared and released imprints in my lower chakras from past sexual experiences (this did not involve touching me at all—in fact, he was several feet away), I swear I could sometimes recognize the person as their energy moved through Nicholas.

He worked by getting me to talk about certain memories or experiences, asking direct and sometimes confrontational questions as he was guided intuitively. This would open the blocked energies in my system, things that had been stuffed away, and he would reach in as if literally grabbing something and pulling it out, making wild noises and contorting his face as the energy shot through him like lightning. I felt the layers of misunderstanding, self-loathing, previous desires for self-destructive behavior, and the opinions of others all falling away. I remember sitting on the couch in his home during my first intensive five-day session and feeling like a child who had just awakened into a twenty-seven-year-old body. *What have I been doing all this time?*

To support my spiritual path and integration of the work we had done, Nicholas suggested I begin a practice called the Latihan. He felt that the Latihan was the practice that kept him clear after his intense work with others. The Latihan is a practice of surrendering to God/dess and the purity of our own souls. Women practice with women and men with men. One is intentionally and ceremonially opened to the Latihan by sitting with a group that is practicing, which creates an "opening" for the connection within the initiate. A palpable energy flows into the space, and the participants are moved by the cleansing energy, sometimes singing, moving, or speaking in tongues. When Nicholas had recommended the Latihan, I felt strongly pulled to follow his guidance.

Jin

Nicholas wanted me to connect with a community of spiritual women, so he introduced me to Jin, who also lived in Los Angeles. I was struggling as my inner world was rapidly changing while my outer world stayed the same, and I had begun to feel suffocated by it. Jin had a charismatic personality and talked openly about her travels and spiritual explorations. She was considerably older than I was, even older than my mother. I wanted her to like me, to approve of me. This desire was the basis of our initial dynamic.

Years went by and we became friends, sharing the practice of Latihan with a wonderful group of women. We traveled together once to visit Nicholas on the East Coast, doing intensive energetic clearing work with each other for three days. Although it felt powerful for me to be with elder teachers, I also felt a bit bullied by Nicholas and Jin. They both wanted to be sure I saw things their way. I didn't see until later that I unconsciously bought into the misbelief that their way was right and they were somehow more attuned to higher guidance than I was. I deferred to them for answers and hesitated speaking what felt true for me.

Nicholas was highly opinionated and would argue with me over friends in my life or guys I was dating if he felt they weren't good for me. I'd always listened to him, until I got into a relationship at age twenty-nine with someone he didn't approve of. I often felt berated by him over this relationship, so much that I took a break for several months from my daily phone calls with him. In these calls, we would check in, I would ask questions, and he would clear me of any unwanted energies I may have picked up throughout the day. As a highly sensitive empath, this was an invaluable support. When I first started seeing clients as a healer, I relied on calling Nicholas after sessions to help me clear any energetic residue. With hindsight, I can see that I set up a pattern of dependency on him.

Years later, I was flattered when Jin wanted to attend my first pilgrimage to Avalon. The following year, she asked to collaborate and colead my next journey with me, one that I was already planning. I knew in my heart that it didn't feel right. I had already put years of work, money, travel, and relationship-building into what I had created, and it was already magnificent. She wanted to incorporate a form of dance she taught, which I'd never really liked, yet I'd always attended her classes to "be a good friend." *Ahh, the pressures I put on myself! Cancer personality and people-pleasing at their height.* Going against my gut feelings, I told myself that I *should* be honored she wanted to collaborate with me—after all, she was my elder, and I would learn a lot.

I did learn a lot, but it wasn't through her teachings. It was through the discomfort and disappointment that I came to reap as a result of the choice I'd made to allow her to collaborate with me. I quickly discovered that she wanted to take what I had created for herself, and she was not willing to share the role of leadership. I experienced her attempting to swoop in and take the stage, standing on the magic and sacredness I had so openly shared with her and claiming it as her own. It felt like a living metaphor of goddess spirituality being dominated and repurposed by patriarchal religion. *The most deceiving part was that her attempts to disempower me were under the guise of intuition and spiritual receiving.* I felt that I had invited a bully into my sacred space.

For example, one day I shared a meditation with her that I felt called to offer the group. Quickly acting as if receiving a strong intuitive message, she said, "Oh no, I'm getting a no on that; that's not good for the group." Her response felt dramatic, and I felt attacked. I explained the significance of the lore of the meditation in connection with the particular place we were in. She then decided she liked the idea, and the previous message she had so strongly received went out the window. Later on, she animatedly preached the story I'd told her that day to the women in the group, without acknowledging she had just learned it from me and disregarding it as something I had intended to share. I began to question her motives, feeling her strong need to be the authority. I started to realize that throughout the years of our friendship, she had continuously given me advice based on these apparent intuitive receptions, which I now was understanding to be heavily influenced by her own desire to be in control.

All of this occurred just days before my first initiation in Avalon, so I didn't have much time to process this awareness before the earthquake of sensing that I had a dis-ease erupted in my consciousness. Jin and I spoke a handful of times before I was diagnosed. We attempted to speak to the shadow material that had emerged for us during the retreat and make peace; however, nothing felt resolved. When the idea of creating a prayer circle was suggested to me, I was already sending group texts to my Latihan circle, which Jin was part of. Something in me knew to be discerning and not include her in the prayer circle; however, the self-defeating cancer personality trait of worrying about being nice and wanting to include everyone won. All of the other women in our shared community were in the group, and I knew it was impossible for her to not find out about it. Around the time the prayer circle was formed, she asked if she could come visit me. I agreed and then regretted it.

It was the third week of my treatment cycle, so I was feeling more like myself, and those days of feeling better were precious to me. She came to see me, her friend who was going through chemo, the one she was seeing for the first time with no hair. Almost instantly, I felt judged, as if I had done something wrong. She didn't ask me how I was doing, hold my hand, offer comfort, or express that she was there to be with me in any way I needed, nothing emotionally or spiritually supportive. She simply charged in and listed the things she thought I needed to do, in her usual demeaning tone that implied I just wasn't good enough as I was and couldn't possibly handle things on my own. She's never had cancer or gone through chemo, and now she's the authority on this, too? When she left, I felt awful.

One evening shortly after I went to look at the What's App prayer circle—receiving messages from my sisters in this group was the best part of each day—I was stunned to see a text across the group chat that read, "Jin left the group." Heat began to rise in my chest. I saw a message explaining that she felt there was an energetic issue with the group so she was departing. She "wished me the best."

How on Earth could she find a problem with a group that's focused on healing, supporting, and sending love to a friend going through cancer? Was she serious? I saw so plainly that she wanted to direct my healing process. The supportive circle of shared sisterhood power, with no leader or hierarchy, did not align with the way she was accustomed to using her energy. I had been allowing, cocreating, and participating in this disempowering dynamic from day one, based on my need for approval. But now, my new teacher—cancer—was calling me forward into a higher level of discernment and personal responsibility.

Chung Fu

During this time of emotional turmoil, I worked with Chung Fu to help me unpack all of the material that was arising as a result of Jin's intrusive negativity. I wanted to hear the response from a teacher who was authentic and true, and who genuinely had my best interests at heart. Chung Fu has ascended from the physical realm, so he has a very different perspective, which I experience as vast and expansive. He is not limited by the constructs of physical-world reality.

I shared my distress with Chung Fu: "When I was trying to let go of the story of betrayal with Jin and all of the things associated with it, I was able to see clearly three women who, in this life, have been a trigger and a betrayal in my process and in my healing journey. It was powerful to realize that they were 'playing their part' perfectly, by walking out of my life during this time when I was so vulnerable. These incidents are bringing up some powerful healing for me."

Chung Fu: Yes, this is part of the gift you are receiving from your growing self-awareness and strength. You are releasing those who are not genuinely with you. Tell me about the others.

"One was a dear friend who had been a close friend for a long time. She was with me the night I was diagnosed, and after that, she didn't call or check in for over a month. I received one brief text message from her several weeks later, once I was already in the trenches of chemo, that felt painfully disengaged and distant. She's completely abandoned me in this process, and I've had a lot of feelings about this. We've been friends for fifteen years.

"Another woman, who is a healer, was very present at the beginning, offering to help me, to be there for me, to be a part of my healing process. She actually charged me money to support me with my nutrition and other things I might need. Then she didn't follow through, and this caused me much more stress than support. At this point, I have chosen not to put any further energy on these situations. But these three women, the two I just mentioned and Jin, who were very much present before my diagnosis, have now become part of a 'removal' process, a clearing out of relationships that no longer serve my highest good."

Clarification and tie cutting are essential when you're dealing with so much. You have to economize on your emotional output. If you look back, you are now able to see that you have been feeding those relationships quite a lot of your energy. You can see the pattern.

But you can't do this anymore. You are no longer able to gloss over these unhealthy relationships. You can no longer afford to use any extra energy to make things alright, and you don't have any emotional energy left to tolerate the situation. You're left with the raw feeling, the raw situation, and that's one of the offerings of this cancer presence. Cancer can be a very uncouth and rude presence. It takes no prisoners; it's just out for the kill. It's going to show you—in a very raw, sometimes brutal, way—whatever it shows you. As scary as this may sound, it's good. But you must follow through and take care of yourself, and really seal off the wound.

So, when you've cut ties, carefully bring yourself back and put a shield up. Because when someone has had access to you, even though you're thinking, "Well, they're not getting in touch, and they're not following through," their karma is coming up. There can be negative energy coming at you from these folks because you've seen them on the inside.

Being seen at that level is very uncomfortable. You might find that when you cut ties, to protect yourself, there might be an attempt on their part to return. That's alright. It might not happen, but if it does, then you're well prepared, and you don't take up the bait. You see it, and you're polite, but you don't reestablish a deep friendship. You keep it at the level of an acquaintance, if at all. In your very tender and exposed state, while you're healing from all of this, you can only have those who are 100 percent trustworthy close to you.

I resonated so deeply with Chung Fu's interpretation of this scenario. My over-giving and people-pleasing tendencies had given extra energy to these relationships that had prevented me from experiencing them clearly. Now that I was depleted and had no choice but to focus solely on myself, the truth was exposed. They were not supportive relationships and probably hadn't been for quite some time. My issue of wanting everything to be friendly and okay had prevented me from seeing things as they were. Cancer, the truth serum, was showing me my role in this.

I knew from my past work with clearing energy that when we have had a relationship, there's an energetic link. This link is fed from the connection and can continue to be fed even years after being in regular contact. This is why energetic hygiene is so important. Chung Fu was speaking about consciously cutting the cord, or tie, and retrieving this much-needed energy for myself. When this is done, the person on the other end, who has become unconsciously accustomed to receiving a charge from you, feels it. They may not understand or know exactly what's happened, but they will think of you and perhaps have the desire to reach out. If this happens, it is a confirmation that the tie cutting has worked. This is why I knew it would not be supportive to respond if any of these people reached out to me at this point.

After Jin left the prayer circle, I was not surprised to hear she called a close friend of mine, one she actually didn't know personally, in an attempt to discuss what was wrong with me and my prayer circle. *It's shocking how a person can make someone else's life crisis about them.* Jin had called Nicholas to tell him about the "negative energies" around me and my prayer group, and asked my dear sister, April, to arrange an intervention call so they could talk to me about this. Now this is something that would have been my absolute worst nightmare in my twenties. To me, they were the authorities on negative energies and in the past, I did everything they said to keep myself clear. What was undeniable about this experience is that I knew with every fiber of my being that they were wrong.

Alisha says, "The biggest authority on you is always you," and I felt the power of my own inner knowing. April told Jin that I was doing better than ever. I was completely empowered and surrounded with pure love, and those who did not see that were not accurately perceiving the situation. I saw with such clarity how the truth of my empowered experience did not at all match or reflect the feedback of these previously trusted spiritual guides. The most ridiculous part is that they were thousands of miles away on the East Coast and completely removed from all of it, trying to tell the friends who were by my side and sitting with me through chemo "how it was." My journey through the sixth gate into the underworld showed me the shadows of beings I had put on a pedestal and given the authority to assess the magic, beauty, and power of my own soul.

INANNA'S DESCENT

Gate 6: Loss of the Lapis Measuring Rod: Spiritual Authority

Inanna enters the sixth gate of the underworld, where her lapis measuring rod is removed from her hand. This rod is a sacred tool used by the gods to measure the truth of souls. It has the power to grant life or death and to command justice. It is connected to the second or sacral chakra, the energy center in the womb of a woman and the hara (belly) of a man. This center governs all one-on-one relationships and the emotions connected to them. Inanna is stripped of the authority she has placed upon this tool, from the energy and power granted by something outside of her.

It's easy to assign power and authority to people outside of ourselves, bypassing the more challenging path of radical personal responsibility for our lives, choices, and our experiences. The stripping of the lapis measuring rod, for me, revealed the shadows within some of my relationships; this was painful, yet necessary in my healing because it directed me to deeper truths within. My compassion for the wounds of others grew as I understood more deeply that we are all navigating our own uniquely complex inner landscape. Inanna and I both journeyed further into the underworld toward the abandoned throne of our own spiritual power and authority.

WISDOM FROM CHUNG FU

"I see the energy of Jin and Nicholas trying to discredit me, cut me down, and disempower me in my journey," I said. "It's noteworthy that it's coming in now because it's part of the energy I'm clearing and letting go of. The powerful thing is that my friend April called to tell me all this (the attempt by Jin and Nicholas at an intervention because I was no longer under their control) had happened, and I wasn't triggered by it. In the past, this would've really upset me, but now I see it for what it is."

Chung Fu: Well, they do their best like any other human being. Sometimes people, even gifted people, develop to a certain point in which their healing power is sufficient to help others, so they go into the field of helping others, but they forget to continue working on themselves. This is very common among teachers and people of the previous generation because there weren't so many alternative healing practices around when they were young. They battled their way through, got to a certain point, and then genuinely believed they were offering the best. If you don't follow what they teach and fall into the mode of that obedient child, they don't have another role to play with you; they don't know what else to do. Because they're not getting fed in the way they're used to, they start to behave in a way that is, underneath it all, quite needy. It's a very subtle, turned-around situation in which they use criticism and a negative reflection of you to get you to say or feel that you need them and come back into the fold. This is the way they receive their own nourishment. It's a quite common hunger or need.

When you cut the ties, ask your prayer circle to put a little protection around you. These teachers are not terrible vampires, but you don't need anything but the powerful energy of love radiating toward you right now. Put up some mirrors and say, "Right now, that energy doesn't empower me. I need only energies that completely support and empower me."

You know cancer is very much part of this journey. The powerful and incredibly confident person you are was seriously undermined in that critical ten to twelve years between your teenage self and your awakening when you realized, "Oh my goodness, I need to wake up and reclaim my life, my power, my being." These teachers came along during that period when you were first waking up.

The beings drawn toward you at that time had very similar patterns, in fact. Strangely enough, just as all the other people who had disempowered you ("do this and do that"; "take these pills") and given you the message that you're a "good girl" only if you listen to them, you went toward that same pattern with these teachers because they appeared to be significantly different from what you'd known. They helped you— that is real, but only up to a point, at which your growing self-awareness resulted in you stepping into your own power. Your growth was their Achilles' heel. But being drawn to them was the best you could do at that time because that's who you were then; that underlying place was in you.

I was resonating so deeply with Chung Fu's assessment of the situation, feeling sparks of insight as many connections were being made inside. "That's exactly right," I replied.

It was time to completely pull all of my energy out of those relationships for good. The voice of my inner guide, teacher, and healer was getting louder. The priestess of old was rising within me, the Lady of the Lake. The veils of illusion within the misperceptions and displacements of power in my relationships were being lifted. Cancer was teaching me that it was imperative I begin making choices from within.

JOURNAL ENTRY, A FEW DAYS AFTER JIN LEFT THE PRAYER CIRCLE

I had such a beautiful vision during prayer circle tonight. Many other circles of light surrounded me, showering me with healing. My prayer circle was there, and then more circles around us; circles within circles and on and on...beaming light and healing that I was directing to my breast. Jin's leaving unblocked something and allowed me to see beyond my previously limited perspective. She was like a shadow in the circle. I felt Lui, Daisy, Luna, friends in Glastonbury and Europe; Mer Horton and friends from childhood; and people from all parts of my life sending light and love. I am so grateful for the way things have unfolded. Thank you for showing me the truth. Blessed be.

PORTION OF A LETTER I WROTE TO JIN, SEVERAL MONTHS LATER AS A HEALING EXERCISE

Being diagnosed with cancer came through an act of pure love and devotion to Goddess in my first dedication. She unearthed what had been hidden in my body. She brought forward ancient material that had been buried deep in my unconscious. She accelerated my path and took me into a direct initiatory experience with Her. The treacherous underworld journey that followed was for me and me alone. It was between Goddess and me. The underworld territory I traversed are depths that can be known only to those who have faced a life-threatening illness.

The assumption that you could have guided me through these places, or that I would have needed you as a conduit to access the wisdom of my own soul's journey, is arrogant and impertinent. The fact that you had your own opinion about what my healing needed to look like for you to participate in the healing circle and support me as a friend is precisely the controlling and disempowering energy I have chosen to release from my life.

What I needed from my sisters was unconditional love and support, and to know they understood that I had all the inner resources necessary to navigate the path I was being asked to walk.

Perhaps through your own lens you saw the group's energy differently than it actually was, and I'm sorry you missed out on the beauty and healing we all experienced.

I was not hurt by you, Jin. I was angry and saddened at the disempowering dynamic I had been in with someone who I thought was my friend. I was hurt by the painful material your actions triggered within me. This was my responsibility and opportunity to heal, and ultimately, it had nothing to do with you.

JOURNAL ENTRY

Today in my vision-journey to Avalon, I sat in the center of the stones at Stonedown. These stones are large; there's a stone altar with an egg stone in the center. The Lady of Avalon spoke to me about Nicholas. I had expressed an old fear and confusion around him being so vigilant about his way to God. He was always testing someone's path and direction, "feeling" if they would go to God or not, and it scared me.

The Lady explained that each individual path of evolution is based on their alignment with their soul's highest purpose; therefore, the direction we go in our learning after each lifetime follows that route. The best we can do is align ourselves with our highest and purest truth, which is exactly what I am doing and will continue to do, and what this year has been about. She said Nicholas was trying to teach me about alignment, although his interpretation was off because he was basing things on his own path as well as coming through his own wounding and abusive communication pattern. Thank you, Lady of Avalon, for explaining this so clearly!

I acknowledge myself for choosing my own higher guidance over that of another.

I honor my own inherent divine protection and trust my alignment with my soul's highest purpose.

Blessed be.

JOURNAL PROMPT

Who in your life do you perceive as an authority figure? Do you defer to them? Where in your life do you give your power away?

MEDITATION

Sit comfortably with your spine straight, or lie down, where you will not be disturbed. Close your eyes, and begin taking in deep diaphragmatic breaths, in through the nose, filling and expanding the belly, and out through the mouth with an audible exhale...ahhh. Repeat three times.

Bring your awareness to your sacral chakra, the energy center that rests a few inches below your naval. Lovingly place your hands there while visualizing the color orange swirling in a circle beneath them.

Bring to mind a person in your life whom you have put on a pedestal or viewed as being in a position of power or authority, and see them standing before you. How do you feel in their presence? Take a moment to scan your body and notice any areas of tightness, observing any feelings or sensations that arise.

Imagine that this person is holding up a mirror. As you look into the mirror, the reflection you see reveals the part of you that has participated in this power dynamic. Allow yourself to receive this image fully. How old is this aspect of you? What fears, wounds, or limiting beliefs are they carrying? How was this aspect of you receiving some form of secondary gain through this relationship, such as validation, security, or a false sense of self-worth?

The perceived authority figure now hands you the mirror. You hold it so that it is now reflecting back at them. This magical mirror reveals the truth behind the authoritative mask, showing you the humanness of this person who carries their own wounds and shadows.

Inanna stands before you at the sixth gate of the underworld, reminding you of the wisdom of your gut feelings and instincts. She asks you to release any false sense of self-worth, security, or validation that you felt you received from this relationship. Allow this energy to flow into the mirror, and when you are ready, hand the mirror to Inanna. She carries it across the threshold of the sixth gate of the underworld, opening you to the understanding that you are the authority of your own life and, therefore, the source of your own deepest truth and inner knowing.

Focus your awareness once again on your hands resting at your sacral chakra, breathing deeply.

Give thanks for the intelligence of your body and the wisdom that it carries.

When you are ready, open your eyes and journal any insights that came forward.

Blessed be.

Chapter Seven

LIVING IN AN UNDERWORLD CAVE

SEVENTH GATE: IDENTITY

"The tree that would grow in heaven
must send its roots to hell."

~ Frederick Nietzsche

"We go down as she goes down
We follow her underground
Hail to Inanna
Who dies to become whole."

~ Suzanne Sterling

RAW TRUTH

I am so sick and tired of the prison that is this bed. My vision is blurred, my head is pounding. I can't think or follow a conversation. I had to turn off a movie the other day because I couldn't follow the story line. I feel persecuted, tortured. Like someone is holding my head underwater and all I can do is struggle to gasp for a moment of air. I feel beaten and punched in the stomach simultaneously.

I have the foulest taste of chemicals in my mouth that never goes away. It's a burning chemical taste that arises from my chest and seers through my mouth in every direction, relentlessly. My eyes water. My nose bleeds. My hands are bright red and raw. I have purple and dark red blisters all over my body, a rare side effect that my doctor has never seen. To combat this, they're giving me steroids, which I loathe. I feel like the gum-chewing little girl in *Willy Wonka and the Chocolate Factory* when she's blown up into a blueberry.

Except I'm a raspberry, crimson and swollen. My head is bald. I can't wait for the day I can burn this dreadful headscarf. I have no eyebrows or lashes. My face and body are swollen and bloated. People assume going through chemo means losing weight, but that's not necessarily true. I've gained twenty pounds, blown up like a balloon from all the steroids they are giving me in an attempt to mitigate more extreme side effects. I don't fit in my clothes or recognize myself in the mirror.

VOICE AUDIO TO PRAYER CIRCLE

Hi, sisters,

I want to put an intention in the space today. This is the first day since starting this round of chemo, light infusion, that I've been able to get out of bed, to sit at my altar, to join our prayer circle. I'm requesting a lot of support for my physical body. I am in a lot of pain, really deep bone aches, like the feeling when you have the flu, but more intense and all over, including all my joints at the same time. In my feet, toes, fingers, ankles, wrists, knees, everything. And my head is pounding.

I know the routine now. Three days after treatment, they give me a shot to boost my white blood cells, and things start getting very intense and overwhelming. My whole body hurts, every muscle, every bone. The touch of my clothes against my skin hurts. Everything hurts. Trying to get into and out of bed is painful because every muscle just aches. Even lightly pressing my finger on my face, or anywhere on my skin, hurts. And then, all the pain morphs into severe aching.

I'm sitting here with my eyes closed because it's too hard to look at the screen. I'm really asking for support from my most human, vulnerable self. In my soul and my heart and my truth, I know this is a spiritual initiation. Yes, I'm walking through the trenches of a massive transformation. And, my human self really needs some support. My human self just needs to say this fucking sucks! Oh, God. It is so hard. I really need to allow myself to say this, and be in this space. Thank you for hearing me.

WHAT IS CHEMO *REALLY* LIKE?

When I first started chemo, I thought I could still continue to live my holistic lifestyle while moving through it, with one foot in both worlds. I was sorely mistaken. Once in the world of chemo, there is no choice but to be fully in it. Everything is affected by this medicine. My stomach lining has changed; the food my body craves—not just craves, but can handle ingesting at all—has changed. While I know weekly acupuncture has greatly supported me because I haven't once vomited or had diarrhea, green juice and salads are a memory of the distant past. I tried to drink wheatgrass at the beginning of chemo and that was probably the sickest I've felt.

I asked my husband to go to the homeopathic pharmacy to get a remedy for nausea, and the woman looked at him point-blank and said, "She needs something for chemo nausea? Nothing here is going to help with that. She needs to smoke pot. Sativa through a vaporizer, that's her best bet." She was stunned to hear I was trying to force down raw foods. "She needs warm, cooked food right now, comfort food."

I remembered sitting with my notebook at my oncologist's office asking about the best diet to support this process and he simply said, "Whatever you can stomach."

I breathed a sigh of relief the day my husband came home with a vaporizer. I realized I had not yet surrendered to this path of medical treatment. If I am choosing this, I must dive in and let it do its work. I must believe in it. It's a short period of time, and I can cleanse and eat raw food on the other side. While I don't have to be limited by the mentality of the paradigm of Western medicine, I can use it as a tool and benefit from the extensive research that has gone into these treatments. And right now, I need all the tools I can get. After my first chemo treatment, I came home with four prescriptions that I had rolled my eyes at, thinking, "Yeah right, I will not take those pharmaceuticals." *I really thought I could do chemo on my terms.*

About two days later, I began suffering from a sensation of a fireball burning in my throat, with painful hiccups and burping, and discomfort even swallowing water. On the day Ryan came home with the vaporizer, I surrendered my resistance and finally tried the heartburn medicine. I had instant relief. I allowed myself to try the rest of the prescriptions they gave me to support the process. I realize that during this period while I am choosing this method of treatment, I have to allow myself the appropriate support to match its strength. Chemo was a short-term solution and I need to go all in. I was incredibly sick and nauseated, and not the kind of nausea that I had ever felt before. This was a chemically induced, claustrophobic kind of nausea from which I felt no escape until I smoked cannabis, which helped me beyond belief. The vaporizer was crucial as I could not have tolerated the smell or taste of smoke. What a powerful medicine cannabis is, and how wrongfully it has been demonized and suppressed.

I changed directions and began allowing myself to eat the foods I craved most, which were comfort foods and the foods I loved as a child. I realized I was feeding and tending to my scared little girl inside as I ingested these foods, and they were helping us both. I'd been strictly gluten and dairy free for many years, and that didn't change. I enjoyed organic, gluten-free, vegan versions of grilled cheese sandwiches, mac and cheese, pizza, and chocolate chip pancakes. I must say, these foods were a source of a lot of comfort! Ryan is a chef and former restaurant owner and lovingly prepared it all for me. Food was a creative expression for him, and he'd plate my "inner kid's meals" beautifully and bring them to me in bed on a tray. When they arrived before me, no matter how shitty I felt, for a moment, I felt like a princess. Recalling his tender support with my meals during this time when food had become such a challenge brings tears to my eyes even now.

MY WITCH'S BREW

One of the most valuable insights I had during treatment was realizing the amount of judgment and self-righteousness present in the new-age community against Western medicine. Using Western medicine is somehow seen as a failure or a cop-out, the misunderstanding being that the "spiritual" way is sticking strictly to natural medicines and holistic treatments. I find this perspective harmful and dangerous; it grossly oversimplifies something extremely complex.

Healing is a deeply personal journey involving many intricate layers. Genetics, blood type, hormone receptors, emotional and spiritual wounds, as well as lessons carried over from past lifetimes and much more that is beyond our understanding all inform what treatment each individual will best respond to. The key to healing lies in listening deeply to our own inner healer, the "still small voice" within, attuning to our inner compass, and allowing the wisdom of the soul—the one who knows the why, where, and how—to lead the way.

When I found out I had cancer, I knew in my bones I had to do chemo. The mixed comments and attitudes I received from people who had never had cancer and did not know what it was like to stand in my shoes were shocking. I felt my defenses go up as if I had to explain myself. *No!* I knew that the cancer personality is people pleasing, needing to be liked and approved of, not wanting to make waves or create conflict, and bending over backwards to accommodate others at the cost of myself and my own truth. I had already suffered from these things terribly. Now, my life depended on my *not* buying into those old patterns.

I knew I had to create my own medicine bag, picking and choosing what felt right for me and tossing what didn't. The key ingredients in my cauldron included: reframing the chemo as light infusions; daily spiritual practice of meditation and visualization; weekly spiritual counseling sessions; shamanic healing during every round (every three weeks); weekly acupuncture and bodywork; flower essences; comfort food; funny movies; episodes of *Grace and Frankie* and *My So-Called Life* reruns; sleeping on an infrared BioMat infused with amethyst crystals; the daily support of prayer circle; the love of Ryan and my family; and lots of cuddles from my magical healing kitties. The brew that was the medicine my soul needed also required a lot of tears, facing fears and deep terror, feeling my feelings, screaming, walking, and being outdoors as much as possible, with bare feet on the earth.

After my third round of chemo, when I felt I was in the belly of the beast, my friends Val and Harmony came over with a shovel. It was raining outside. They dug up rich, beautiful earth and filled a bowl, then lay me on the floor with blankets and buried my feet in the dirt. I rubbed this dirt all over my belly and prayed to Mama Earth to transmute my sickness.

Knowing that I was descending deeper into the physical pain as the cumulative effects of chemo grew stronger, my prayer circle sisters had sent me flowers for every color of the rainbow, starting with red. Every day for eight days I received the most beautiful flowers— red, orange, yellow, green, blue, purple, and white. Looking up from my bed and seeing the rainbow bouquets all lined up will be a vision

I remember for the rest of my life. On this day, with my feet and belly covered in the wet earth, my friends arranged the rainbow flowers in a circle around me. We sat together in silence, breathing deeply. They weren't trying to fix me and didn't need me to say anything. They simply sat by my side and helped me feel less alone.

Experiencing their loving presence, sitting with me in my pain, was truly a gift. Later, I heard from another friend that she had been working with a medicine man while I was in the trenches. He had her do an exercise where she wrote the names of all the people in her life on one piece of paper. After looking at it a moment, he said, "Who's Taylor? She's in the hell realms right now." Hearing this actually comforted me; I felt validated.

HEL IS A NORSE GODDESS

I find it endlessly fascinating how blatantly modern religions are based on pagan underpinnings. Most people don't know that Hel is a Norse goddess of the underworld who presided over the dead. Nearly all churches in Europe were intentionally built over sacred sites that were once dedicated to Goddess, places on the land where the earth energies were palpable. There was no denying the power that existed in these sites, and it was not possible to erase them from the memories of the culture because they had been revered as ancestral places of worship. A patriarchal agenda that had less to do with honoring the Divine than it did with control and suppression, covered, built over, or repurposed these places to harness and manipulate their energies.

As I lie here in bed, I imagine that I am clearing and cleansing away all patriarchal suppression from my body, heart, and spirit. I am releasing all programming and any limiting belief systems or energies I have been imprinted with that involve control and suppression. I let go of all the experiences of being burned at the stake, crucified, or ostracized, including experiences at school as an innocent young girl in which I was put down or made to feel I wasn't smart enough, pretty enough, or that what I had to say wasn't valuable. I'm remembering a conversation with Chung Fu when he spoke of depression as suppressed anger:

You have to expect to meet the place inside you that was given drugs at a young age; you didn't want to take them, but they made you. You became depressed because you weren't allowed to express your feelings, but underneath this, you were actually angry, disappointed, and afraid. You were told to just get on with it and cope. You're a sensitive, a psychic; these inclinations had to be suppressed, as well. This is where the cancer came from. Of course, you were drawn to heal it, but you see, the cancer had already formed. You've been thrown into an even deeper process with your past.

"Are you saying that this feeling I'm having now of being suppressed and having my system worn down by the chemo drugs is bringing up memories of my system being suppressed by Ritalin at age fifteen?" I asked.

Absolutely, dear one. Once you understand what's going on, you'll be better able to get through it, rather than being locked in worry about the treatment while you're also having all of these intense emotions rise up.

Chung Fu's insight into the damaging effects of Ritalin became even more profound when I learned that not only is it classified as a Schedule II substance (which places it in the same category as cocaine and morphine due to its high potential for addiction), a study conducted on children after taking Ritalin for only three months revealed that every child developed chromosome abnormalities, which are associated with increased cancer risk. Chung Fu was speaking to multiple layers of truth, all tracing back to this particular time in my life.

. . .

Goddesses like Hel and Ereshkigal rule the domain of suppressed memories—the ones that have been cast aside, feelings that were shoved away, truths that weren't spoken. To heal, I must go toward them, face them, bring them back to me. They contain my energy, they are part of me, and without them, I am left with little holes in my energy field, like a moth-eaten sweater. I don't have to go far right now; I am already dwelling in the realms of the underworld, with the dark goddesses Hel, Ereshkigal, and Keridwen. I have taken up residence here; my eyes have adjusted to the dark. My awareness has dropped down so deep within me that I've gone through a black hole, through a portal into the land of the dead.

As I walk through the seventh gate of the underworld, I am stripped bare, naked, and raw. There is nothing left to protect me, no layers to cover the truth of my being. I am as I am. I am surrendered to the perfect ways of the underworld. I am naked as the day I was born, once again on the threshold between life and death, between matter and spirit, between the seen and the unseen. I am facing all the things that have separated me from my original innocence and purity. I must allow these things to die if I want to live.

INANNA'S DESCENT

Gate 7: Stripped of Her Robe: Identity

As Inanna walks through the final gate of the underworld, she is stripped of her last remaining garment, her robe. She is naked. To face her dark sister, Ereshkigal, she must be stripped of anything that has kept her identified with the life she has lived before this moment. Inanna must die to everything she has been and shed the layers of the existence she has known so that she may truly meet her shadow, the place of her power. Ancient pagans practiced rituals and ceremonies in the nude as a way of representing the purity of one's being, releasing the trappings of the world. Nakedness was seen as a way to feel closer to the Divine.

For Inanna to know the truth and power of her own divinity, she had to be stripped of everything. The seventh gate of the underworld is associated with the root chakra, our place of survival, safety, tribe, and origin. When Inanna faces Ereshkigal, she faces death, surrendering the life she has known. Lifeless, she hangs on a hook for three days and three nights.

PERSONAL MEDITATION

In my meditation, I journeyed to the barren wasteland of the Western Isle of the Dead, which is one of Avalon's names. Avalon shows us our shadows and helps us retrieve and heal the lost or disowned aspects of ourselves. Within Avalon, there are many dimensions and realms of experience. I'm beginning to understand the land of the dead as a realm that holds our shadows, rather than being a barren realm for the departed. The wasteland is also the consequence of a world that doesn't honor Goddess: a barren earth. When I see Blue in Avalon, in my visions, he is vibrant and in beautiful, lush landscapes. He is not cast away in a barren place.

When I journeyed to the barren wasteland, I was a large, ancient, white-and-tan bird with a rounded head. I've seen these birds in my visions lately, in the past life regression work with Jim George. In these memories, I am on the Isle of Avalon and merging my consciousness with these particular birds to go on journeys and shape-shift.

Today, I could feel myself flying. I felt the cool air and mist off the ocean against my skin. The ocean was a deep, dark blue, and I saw a whale spouting. I felt the heat of the sun as I flew closer to the barren wasteland. I came to a scraggly tree, and to my dismay, I saw my left breast hanging on the tree, along with an ancient-looking silver dagger with carvings on it. I saw a dark blue, magical-looking cloak with embroidery and symbols around the sides, and a golden aura emanating from it. I felt the energy of my childhood pony, Misty, and saw a photo of her hanging there. I saw a pair of little girl's white cotton underwear. I saw the ring that my ex-boyfriend proposed to me with when I was twenty-eight. I thought, "Oh no, what is that doing here?" I saw a beautiful, elaborate piece of bronze jewelry that was like a breastplate that could fit over my heart and adorn my chest.

I shape-shifted from the bird's perspective back to my human form, and my left breast just seamlessly integrated onto my body, surrounded with light. I felt a sigh of relief and heard, "I am whole." I put on the underpants and felt that I was restored to my original innocence. All of this gave me a sense of being uplifted and powerful. I felt healed. Sexual wounds dissipated and I felt completely pure. I placed the dagger near my right hip, tucked away in a little belt, and put the cloak on, which felt very natural. Misty, my pony, went into my heart and that felt right; she is a part of my heart. I put the beautiful jewelry on my chest; it felt regal and tribal.

The ring was the last thing left, and I felt that I had never given it a proper burial. I needed to consciously bury it with love and respect instead of casting it away into nothingness. In my mind, I dug a hole in the earth and lovingly buried it, pouring sacred water over it. Placing my hands on the earth, I spoke these words: "I give thanks for this path that I did not choose." I then stood and felt the sun on my face and said, "I give thanks for the path that I did choose and the one I am choosing. Blessed be."

SESSION WITH CHUNG FU

"Physically, I am halfway through treatment," I said. "I've had three light infusions, and I have three more to go. This last round was especially difficult, the most challenging so far. My acupuncturist told me it's very common for the third round to be really hard. The first two rounds, you're still pulling from the reserves in your body, but by the third, you're more depleted, so it's more taxing. I found myself going to a pretty dark place. I felt exceptionally sad and couldn't stop crying for days. Usually I'm comfortable emoting, and expressing, and releasing, but the depth of despair and sadness I was feeling was overwhelming. It brought on an uncontrollable release of tears. This time, it took me longer to recover; this was just a lot harder.

"My hormones have plummeted. They're giving me a Lupron shot to essentially make my body think I'm in menopause to protect my fertility. The drug suppresses my ovaries so there's no cellular activity around my womb, and that, by default, creates a protective barrier so the chemo doesn't go to my ovaries or womb. The side effect is that my hormones have completely plummeted, so I'm feeling the effects of the suppression or lack of hormones. I'm having intense hot flashes and feel very dry."

Chung Fu: When you find yourself in those deep and despairing places, just let go. It sounds like you're doing this really well already. Think of it as an endurance test—your power is great enough to deal with it, but you have to let it flow through you. Tears are good. What else are you doing to support yourself physically?

"I'm feeling very supported with acupuncture. But the first ten days after the treatments, I'm extremely fatigued and emotional. My head hurts, and I find it hard to read or focus my eyes. While I feel like it would really support me to read an uplifting book or listen to a meditation, I find it challenging to do those things after the light infusion. I often end up watching funny movies because I'm trying to lift my spirits. I'm wondering if you can suggest anything else I can try to make myself feel better?"

Enjoying comedy is probably the very best thing you can do. That's coming from your higher Self. Chemo alters brain function; you can't really protect yourself against that. It dulls functions of the brain and messes around with synapses and neurons. The result is that you don't recognize your own thoughtforms. You don't recognize what's inside your head. It's not what you put there. All your attention is going into resisting and not believing in any of those negative, painful thoughts that are happening subliminally in your mind. When you have less conscious control, the subconscious takes over.

If you can, engage the subconscious mind with jokes and frivolous trivia. Really, I mean stupid things. Don't even worry about whether it's intelligent enough for you. Don't worry. Just be a child. Watch cartoons. It doesn't matter because you're just finding the best ways to handle the fact that you can't think like you usually do. This is not you; it's your actual physical brain. There's no point in taxing it and trying to force it to do something you'd prefer. Those abilities will come back. You and your brain will bounce back. This is a side effect of the chemo.

Ask yourself: What do you feel inside? What do you want? Do you want to have a bath? Do you want to go for a little walk? Do you want to see something humorous or something beautiful? Perhaps a fashion show? Just feel into what would be fun because it can get pretty hard after a while to find anything fun. If you can, just accept what makes you feel good without judgment. From where I sit, you're doing this hard work pretty well.

Everything is dulled down, like you've been struck by a meteor. Your body has been slammed by the impact of the collision. It's not easy to believe that you'll recover, but you just have to give yourself time. You have to remind yourself that it's just another couple of months, just three more infusions. Tell yourself, "I'm just going to get through this." Accept any amount of bodywork, hugs, cuddles, and foot massages, anything that gives you sensory pleasure. You do need help, dear one.

You're being beaten up right now. Violent energy is entering your system. You need soothing—especially feminine hands or gentle love from Ryan. Soothing love.

Allow yourself to accept the fact that this is traumatic. Don't pretend it's not happening. You're dealing with some very deep past-life and early childhood disturbance, as well, which, in a way, you can't quite deal with yet. That will happen after the treatment. You'll be able to go in with your big-power self, eventually, and deal with the actual underside of it all.

Chung Fu's words were, in themselves, soothing. I needed to hear the hope they contained, and I also needed to be reminded that my body was under siege from the chemo. I closed my eyes and placed one hand on my heart and one over my womb, inwardly promising to be even more gentle with my body, especially my brain. I had to trust in the healing that was occurring and know that I would be resilient on the other side. I felt relief as I welcomed the familiar sensation of cool tears flowing over my hot, swollen cheeks, letting go over and over again.

You go into despair and crying because, as the treatment lessens your outer strength, it also affects your inner spirit muscles, so your feelings come rushing up. This includes the seed from which these feelings originally began—a lack of support from the feminine—which allowed the illness to develop. You felt "given away" by your mother, like, "Well, you're just giving me away to all these other people and none of them understand me. I don't feel safe." This is the core feeling underneath your trauma.

"Yes," I replied. "For the first time, this all really clicks. I'm actually accessing that feeling of being given away, the unmothered place, the deep sadness of being sent away, the feelings of being so alone as a teenager. The whole line of energy around this piece of my past has anchored, and I feel it—and understand it—in a much deeper way."

Also realize it wasn't just that your mother sent you away and you felt the loss of that love and the safety of her embrace. The drugs sent you away, as well. This is a really big revelation, isn't it? It's as though you said, "I'm just going to wait over here, and I'm not going to do that life that isn't mine."

So, depression—and the sense of feeling strange, estranged from people, and unable to fully connect—showed up. You felt kind of outlawed and exiled. Even though, physically, you were still at the schools, somewhere you were coping with very old feelings, even from other lives. Layers and layers of repression stacked up in your womb center and sent messages to your body that things were not right.

As you activated your priestess self and came into these memories, your body was telling you that you needed to find out, "What's going on in here?" From your inner work, there has been, luckily, an acceleration of your awareness and your ability to follow through to discover what's going on.

There's a sense of urgency about this, all brought about by this journey. The priestess was there when you were twelve years old, and she's in a hurry now. She understands that if you don't figure this out, it's a threat to her life—to your life. Your soul knows: all of this matter has to clear for you to be a priestess. So, it has all been brought forward. What I'm really saying to you is that your healing journey, in a certain way, accelerated the manifestation, and all of your feelings of repression and anger have actually come into a form.

Now that you are aware of your trauma around losing the mother-connection, of being "given away," along comes a fear that this kind of rejection will repeat. When you're not fully yourself, no matter how much your friends or your partner express love, you don't feel you're worthy of love. You go to that place of, "Maybe they're going to leave me. Maybe they're going to give me away, too." The panic is in the place of being loved. In fact, you could even say that because they're expressing love for you, you don't feel like yourself. Your inner equation says, "I give the love. I'm the one in power. I'm the one who gives the love." You don't feel like yourself when this equation is turned upside down.

Your sacred, primal relationship was with your mother, but she didn't hear you. So, now when you're in your primary love relationships that are also sacred love, you don't feel safe. But ultimately, this is about you not feeling safe with yourself.

Don't expect miracles while you're going through the treatment. Don't push yourself. Just listen to me a little bit and take it in, but don't think, "I have to fix this straightaway. I can't allow this to go on." Don't think like this because this isn't you. This is the powerful drug that is running through your body and having its physical and mental effect on you. While it's doing its work, it's wiping out some of your functions, as well. Remember that the light infusion has to be as powerful as the cancer to meet it on its own ground.

This is the dis-ease of your time. Cancer challenges you to come fully back into your power. As someone on a spiritual journey, it can be hard to believe this because of the way the drugs make you feel. You must give it some time and understand that this is the undoing of an energy that's gotten into your place of power—or rather, it's gotten into where your power wasn't in your body.

"I am so thankful that you framed it that way," I said. "I've been relating to this experience as an initiation, a reclamation of my full self, and an awakening into my power. I'm realizing I had high expectations that I would harness all the gifts and blessings by the end of chemo. I understand that you're saying this is a process. Part of it is the physical wiping out of the dis-ease and part of it is getting in touch with and working on the psychic trauma of being given away along with releasing past life trauma. I haven't been holding this as a process of 'undoing.' I've been thinking that if I'm not completely healed by the end of chemo, I will have failed."

There's no pretending with the light infusion. The chemo is a very powerful means of disabling cells that have a stronghold on your body. While it does its duty wiping out unwanted dis-ease, the rest of the body, unfortunately, has to temporarily suffer through some earth-shattering side effects. Keep reminding yourself that this part is temporary, and there are some good, new therapies to help with this. Your pituitary and pineal glands are affected, meaning that your power of calling in your higher Self and using your visioning powers is diminished. But let this go, as I've said. These things will return. Be like a child watching movies. Laugh as much as you can. Cry, but don't get attached to crying. Don't be angry with yourself if you're exhausted and all you can do is flop around from bed, to bath, to chair. Just get through it.

You're living in a toxic, drug-induced environment, and you have to rest. You're not being energized; you're being depleted, for a purpose. Medicine and science haven't yet figured out how to treat you without depleting the whole system. You have a strong body, mind, and spirit. Right now, the strength of your chi, of your actual energy field, is dumping you into your emotional sublayer, and you don't have your usual strength to deal with it. Meditations are hard to follow right now because they are aimed at activating the pineal and pituitary, and working with those centers. This is too much for you at this time; you just can't be bothered. Your body is completely obsessed with trying to track what on Earth is going on.

Chung Fu's words washed over me, his wisdom always bringing a sense of peace. I imagined I was holding myself as a child. She is around age five, wearing overalls and a purple turtleneck with tiny holes in it from the claws of the kitten in her arms. She and I both feel so happy being with animals. I realized how much I—we—needed to be seen, the both of us, and to be understood by others. I vow to see and understand her, honoring the ways she needs to be comforted as we move through this.

Your brain, your subconscious, and all of your inner muscles of think-ing—automatic thinking, body thinking, and emotional thinking—are trained on one thing: What is in my body? What is this? Cancer is silent, which is why it's so dangerous. You don't even know it's in your body. But chemo is a loud energy that's actually matching the cancer, meeting it, and facing off with it. You can "hear" this. It's important that you're as relaxed as possible and that, in a sense, you go along with it. It may become increasingly difficult to see the chemo as a light infusion, but continue visioning it in just this way, like you did with the very first treatment.

TONGLEN: A HEALING PRACTICE TO RESTORE MY LIFE FORCE

While Inanna is in the underworld, her devoted servant comes to her aid, giving her sacred water and nourishment to bring her back to life. My healing circle came to my aid with the healing practice of Tonglen, which Chung Fu suggested I add to my medicine bag:

Tonglen is an old Tibetan practice in which one person who has asked for healing sits in the center of a circle, either physically or ethereally, surrounded by friends who are willing to offer support. This is a prac-tice of sending and receiving, and the vehicle is the breath. The one in the center practices breathing out her pain, releasing it to the circle. Those in the circle visualize taking in the pain of the one in the center and sending it back into the earth. Then, those in the circle drink up the earth's energy and send that fresh, clean-energy breath back to the one who needs healing, who accepts the return of the cleansed breath.

The one in the center must be ready and willing to receive healing. The repetitive breathing in and breathing out is about relaxing, letting go, taking a free breath, and breathing out again. The group focuses on the one in the center, drawing any darkness from this person's breath through their own body, letting go of it through their lower body centers and releasing it into the earth. They may make sound, or just breathe out. They breathe new energy in, filling up and sending that fresh energy to you. In their mind's eye, they draw off heavy, negative energy and send it down into the Great Mother's belly. Then, they draw back the power of Mother Earth, filling up with it, and sending it to the one they are supporting. Do you think you've got the hang of this?

I was definitely ready to receive extra support and life-force energy. I was concerned about my friends absorbing the energy that was coming from me, and Chung Fu assured me of the inherent protection that comes with working with the healing power of the earth. Mother Earth is doing the work, the energy flowing into her for transmutation with purified energy returning.

Imagine your friends as pipes. They are attached to you, pulling off dark energy and sending it into the earth, then drawing up the chi— and the life force—and sending it to you. This is a very primal breath practice. It's a very specific concentration practice that requires a little bit more attention than other practices, and therefore, the energy that is exchanged is quite strong. Don't worry about whether you are in rhythm with the group. Just breathe in the light coming from your friends, up from the earth. You can do this simultaneously or at the same time, or with alternate breaths. You're receiving the light and expelling the hurting, painful, negative energy.

JOURNAL ENTRY

Just trying to record some of my feelings while I am feeling them. The intensity of this experience is so severe, I often feel like someone is holding my head underwater and I am gasping for air. I'm in the darkest depths of the underworld, in the mud, my head submerged, and I'm fighting my way out. I don't even know how to describe the depth of despair, pain, and fogginess I am existing in. I see my friends traveling, going on vacation, living a normal life. Everyone's been talking about astrology lately and Mercury retrograde. To me, that feels like such a luxury—to be concerned only with everyday problems! To worry only about the ebb and flow of your emotions, monthly cycles, and PMS! What a joy! That feels so light and free. Such a privilege. Honestly. To be healthy. To feel all of those things. I know with such conviction that after this, I'll have a different perspective on how to live the rest of my life, and I'm grateful for this. I will always maintain a deep appreciation for life, health, and the blessings all around me. I am not afraid of anything anymore! I am going to seize life—dive in!

DREAM JOURNAL ENTRY

Dreamed I was sleeping in a bear cave. I was hibernating to restore my strength. The cave had paintings on the walls that looked like they were from Neolithic times. There were symbols carved in the stone. I was restoring my strength; it was beautiful. In another part of the dream, my eyesight was so blurry I couldn't see. Everything was gray and white like a fuzzy TV screen. My sight is changing.

DREAM JOURNAL ENTRY

I'm traveling on a boat with two others, going to an island. I'm banishing and exorcising ghosts. I'm sitting on a bed in my underwear and a bra that is unhooked and hanging loosely over me. I am speaking commands to banish these ghosts. I hear loud banging and clamoring noises, as everything is falling down.

JOURNAL PROMPT

What does it mean to you to be naked? When was a time in your life that you felt exposed and vulnerable? Who would you be without all the external identifications and trappings of the outside world?

MEDITATION

Sit comfortably with your spine straight, or lie down, where you will not be disturbed. Close your eyes, and begin taking in deep diaphragmatic breaths, in through the nose, filling and expanding the belly, and out through the mouth with an audible exhale...ahhh. Repeat three times.

Visualize your breath flowing down your spinal column, from the nape of your neck to the base of your spine. Imagine your breath exhaling through your root center at the base of your spine, between your legs. As the power of the breath increases in this area, see the energy center of your root glowing the color red. This center governs your sense of survival, safety, and primal nature, as well your connection to the earth, tribe, and origins.

See Inanna standing before you, at the entrance to a cave. She is asking you to remove your clothing, jewelry, and watch—anything you are wearing on your body. If you have any tattoos, imagine they are dissolving from your skin in Inanna's presence. She asks you to contemplate the meaning you have given these things in your life, reminding you that when you first came into this world, you were naked as you are now.

Inanna collects the items that previously adorned your body. Now that you are completely free and unencumbered, she invites you to walk with her into the cave. This cave is a place of surrender, release, and rebirth.

As your eyes adjust to the dark, notice what you see here in this cave. Perhaps a memory, an animal, a person or guide; maybe you notice painting or carving on the walls. Trust what impressions you receive.

Take some time to be with whatever is here for you.

When you are ready, bring your hands to your low belly and come back to your breath, sending it down to the base of your spine.

Scan your body and notice if anything has shifted internally. How do you feel?

Give thanks for whatever has taken place in this cave, for it is in service to your healing and liberation.

Slowly open your eyes and journal any insights that came forward.

Blessed be.

Ascent

SEVEN GATES
OF
RECLAMATION

Chapter Eight

RETRIEVAL

SEVENTH GATE: CHOOSING LIFE

"The cave you fear to enter holds the treasure you seek."

~ Joseph Campbell

Living in my underworld cave for many months opened gateways to deep pockets of wisdom and memory within my soul. There were no veils of separation, no psychic interference, no distractions from the outside world. I was in the void, in the cosmic womb. I was in the place of birth and death, experiencing myself as the great mystery.

After receiving my diagnosis, my aunt introduced me to a healer named Jim George, a quirky, gentle, magical man I immediately recognized on a soul level as a teacher from a past lifetime. Jim had practiced hypnotherapy for many years; being in his presence quickly dropped me into a deep state of peace and equanimity. We worked with a technique he'd developed called "stillness," a process of quieting the brain to resonate at 7.83 hertz, also known as the Schumann frequency, which is the vibration emitted from Mother Earth's heartbeat. When the brain is resonating at 7.83 hertz, cellular healing and regeneration occurs, which is why spending time in nature, particularly barefoot, feels restorative.

During my sessions with Jim, most of which were over the phone, I would drop into a place of serene calmness, and from this state, Jim would assist me in shining a light into the dark caverns of my underworld cave, illuminating soul memories in a clear, visceral, experiential way. Some of what I experienced could have been described as past-life regression; however, Jim encouraged me not to relate to it from a linear perspective. I was remembering everything that came up from the past in the present moment.

VISION, WHILE WORKING WITH JIM GEORGE

I visited Avalon, where I was a teacher. This came forward in an expansive way, beyond anything that could be captured in stories, myths, or legends. The woman I perceived as the Lady of the Lake was the priestess attuned to all energies at once.

. . .

I am in a cave sitting before an altar with carved tools. I see a wooden object, shaped like a spoon with a spiral carved around its edges. The object is wider toward the bottom circle, and the top is pointed. I use this instrument for writing symbols into the earth/dirt/sand to teach. There is a dagger on my altar and a few other carved wooden tools.

I am teaching thirteen maidens in my cave. I am drawing symbols that transmit the frequencies of the four energies—air, fire, water, and earth. We do not call them "elements," but instead work with them as part of the web of energies in which we cohabitate and with which we cocreate. All of Earth's creatures—the trees, birds, stones, animals, air, fire, and water—have their own specific vibratory signature. I understand all of these innately and create symbols for them that hold an energetic signature or transmission. I use these to teach my students. We do not manipulate energy. There is a way we work with energy in complete communion with the Divine and with a knowledge and respect for the ultimate power of Divine will, above all.

On this day, we are preparing for a ceremony, an important rite of passage for the maidens. It is a test for them to demonstrate all they have learned. I am tuning into their level of integrity in their practices, although they are unaware of this. I am feeling into the purity of their devotion. I am standing in the center of a large stone circle wearing a heavy crown with antlers on my head. I feel soft bands of animal fur wrapped around my wrists and ankles, and a deerskin over my body. All the maidens are proceeding up a hill to the stones. They enter the circle one by one and each takes her place in front of a stone.

We begin a series of movements to open the gates...we are opening a bridge/portal to a sister island we work closely with. The tribe there is in ceremony with us; they are drumming and holding a grounding earth energy. There is an etheric white bridge of light. We are spiraling around in a circle in one direction and the birds are flying in a circle overhead in the opposite direction...clockwise and counterclockwise. We are creating a vortex. The maidens merge their consciousness with one of the birds and travel across this bridge to the sister island and back again.

I am in the center of the stones and I am huge, taller than all the stones. My awareness is everywhere—with all my students as well as on both islands. There are three islands that work together, creating ceremonies according to different times of the year. They are Avalon, Iona, and the Isle of Mona. There are still portals to Avalon alive in these places today: modern-day Glastonbury, Iona, and Anglesey, Wales.

As I come out of this vision, I see the ancient triple spiral symbol that is seen in Neolithic art, and I understand it to be an illustration of these rituals, the spiraling of energies to open the vortex portal, and the three islands.

SOUL RETRIEVAL

Soul retrieval was a significant theme during the course of my healing journey. Sometimes during times of distress, aspects of the soul may dissociate from the body and energy field. The absence of this energy can lead to confusion, depression, addiction, or dis-ease. The source of this separation may come from childhood or beyond this life, as the consciousness of the soul holds imprints and memories from other lifetimes. Soul retrieval is a term used to describe a method of shamanic work. This work involves journeying into the memories through the core of the heart, the three realms (the upper, middle, and lower worlds), and past timelines or other dimensions where a piece of that soul may be stuck to heal sources of trauma and spiritual pain and invite the departed energy to return.

Retrieving and reintegrating these pockets of soul energy from other lifetimes or experiences is essential for our health and wholeness. In my quest to heal at the deepest level possible, I was seeking to know the origins of my pain, of the dis-ease. I desired to retrieve and reclaim any parts of my energy that had been separated from me, from any time across the expanse of my soul's voyage. My strong intention to heal at the deepest level guided my journey, bringing into my conscious awareness what needed to be seen and remembered from this life and others. The experiences and memories that arose brought me an expanded sense of understanding, and I had many moments of profound peace, wonderment, and awe at the beauty and intricacy of the divine plan.

As I journeyed further down the path of soul retrieval, the living blueprint of this plan emerged through my inner senses of seeing, knowing, feeling, and hearing. The voices of the lost ones I had once been went from distant whispers to thunderous reverberations through my being. Their calls echoed from the walls of my underground cave and grew louder and clearer as I welcomed them home, filling me with their power. Their sounds and frequencies began to unify and harmonize with one another, creating a beautiful melody that resonated as one soul song, singing me into wholeness.

SESSION WITH CHUNG FU: BECOMING ONE WITH THE LADY OF THE LAKE—CLEANSED WITH THE WATER OF LIFE

Chung Fu: As you walk in the Isle of Avalon, the priestess self you're retrieving is walking toward you from another part of the isle. She is looking for you as you're looking for her. She is walking on the land, deep within the inner planes of Avalon. As you walk, the first thing you come to is the lake. You walk into the lake. You are wearing a long gown made of sacred cloth, and you are wading out into the lake. As you wade out, the Lady of the Lake comes and says, "Come with me." Effortlessly, she brings you to her boat.

"I will take you," she says. "I will be your ferry person today. Come, in my special barge, and we will cross the lake. I will take you to where your priestess self has been with me all this time, waiting for you."

As you step into her barge, you experience an ecstatic feeling. Like being carried to heaven. The barge floats effortlessly across the lake. The Lady of the Lake is directing it with her will. All the while, her kind eyes are searching deep within you. She is like your mother, but she is also you. As you approach the shore and the Isle of Avalon, deep feelings rise up within you. Remembering, remembering.

As the boat comes to shore, she steps out first and holds out her hand to you. You step out, once again wading through the waters, coming to the shore of the beach. Many are there waiting to greet you, and more and more appear. For when the Lady brings one back with her, they know it is of great importance. All of the sisters and the brothers, those who have been priests and priestesses, those who have walked their lives, know what that is like upon the Earth. They are keen to hear your stories. They are linking arms with you, gathering around you.

The Lady walks in the center, and the whole group walks on up the beach, up the shore, toward the woodlands, where the cool shade embraces you. The trees whisper in the breeze, and many little beings peek out of hideouts, homes, and the woodland landscape. As you walk, they are excited, whispering and listening. Oh, they know a great deal, and they knew you were coming. The Lady told them, and they have prepared a ceremony for you. "We know how you have been suffering," they say. "We have been sending you love, energy, and healing. We know that you have felt us. We love you with all our hearts."

By the time you're inside the woodland, there are many creatures walking with you. Birds in the trees and in the stream that runs all around the Isle of Avalon. You feel yourself drawn to walk in that stream, which runs down to the lake, fed from high up on the mountain. The Lady guides you and shows you, and all your brothers and sisters join you as you walk upstream, up and up. The woodland carries on and on, upward, up the mountain. Then, you just want to lie down, as the stream cascades around you, cleansing you as this spirit water from deep inside the Western Isle pours through you. This stream of life links the inner world with the outer world, linking you to the source of your being.

Up, up you climb to the waters, refreshing your feet, splashing on your body. All your friends are with you. Some are walking in the stream behind you. Some to the side. The Lady walks ahead, leading you up and up. Occasionally, she looks back, smiles. You begin to see the birds circling, flying in the blue sky above. The trees and the grassy mountainous terrain reveal themselves. A stream starts to flow around the sidewalks. You look down and can see a crevice as you are climbing. At this place, she beckons to you and takes you to where the stream forms to a beautiful small pool that shines in the sun that sparkles on the water. She beckons to you to lie down in this beautiful, clear pool of blue, pure water. She beckons to all your sisters and brothers to stand around you as you bathe.

"This is my birthing pool," she says. "I have called you here on this day to bathe you in my womb waters, in my mountain belly."

You realize that around you, the mountain carries on a little. The top is a little further away, and you're in this beautiful, central dip. The waters here feel very safe and healing. As you bathe in the waters, you become aware of a group of beings a little further away, moving toward you. As you look more closely, you recognize a being who is you. She is the priestess, who came here to return to you. She came to reconnect, heal, and listen.

As the group approaches, you rise from the water, as though the Lady is in you and with you. You walk out a little bit, welcoming this group to join you, standing opposite this beautiful, tall being. She's in shining white that shimmers. You look down at yourself, and you see that you are also in white.

She has big tears in her eyes as she remembers her Earth life. She sees and remembers the pain you have been carrying. She looks at you with great compassion and love, and you return the same look to her. This is like looking into a mirror. The magnetism grows and grows as you get closer and closer until you are facing each other, touching. The love is intense, big, and strong. The Lady is in you both, as though you are two aspects of each other. It's as though she's speaking from within you.

"My beloved. My most beloved, with whom I have walked. I have brought you together to unify you. May the power be reborn fully, on Earth."

She calls you both on the inside to join together. "My beloveds. You have been separated by time and memory. It is time now to be one

again. One being. With the full power of your soul. You can now
return to Earth."

She continues to speak as if from within you. Your bodies get so close,
they become one body melding one into another. Her body is so full
of energy, light, love, and power. It infuses you with a fresh, young
strength. You can hear the words, "I love you. I love you. I love you. I
love you," and you are not sure if it is the Lady or your priestess self, for
you have become one.

"We are the love; we are the one. We are the love; we are the one love.
We are one: one being, one love."

Inside, you can feel her, your beautiful priestess self, breathing into
every cell: her life force and her healing power. As this moment of
ecstatic unity happens, it's as though all of the brothers and sisters are
drawn really close. The sound lifts up from all their hearts: of joy, cele-
bration, the retrieval, of reuniting with them.

The goddess leads you back into the pool of one being, uniting, being
born again from her womb pool of pure, blue, light water. She sings her
song. Let it come through you. Let her unite you in your body—just
feel her. In whatever way—in words, sound, or silence—feel her. From
deep in her soul, love.

At this moment, I felt filled up with light and love, the kind that is
not directed toward one person but instead toward the entire world.
The kind that overrides personal pain and struggle and holds sacred
appreciation for the gift of this life. From deep within my heart, I
began to sing a song that has no words, a song of joy.

As the light pours down, blessing you, lighting up the water and shin-
ing deep into your body, feel the multidimensionality. Feel the many
dimensions of beauty pouring in from the water, from the land, from
the air, from the sun. Drink in the presence of the Lady of the Waters.

All the brothers and sisters are making offerings, wearing petals, herbs, flowers, and bringing their offerings to you, as you are reborn in the womb of the Lady, in her deep mountain belly.

They bless you, and they bless your path, as you feel the strength and power of she who has returned. On the inside, you feel the layers of power returning to your body, to your priestess self, who has suffered. And who, like you, are returning from the suffering to live again, to be reborn into the fullness of her being. To embody the goddess on her sacred land. Feel the Lady of the Lake as she fills you and your whole body with her loving presence. Fills your heart, and fills your mind with your visions that are her visions, your dreams that are her dreams, your creations that are her creations. Drink in the waters of her emotional power to sustain you through the long Earth walk of manifestation, knowing you can return to refresh, to regenerate, to uplift yourself. You can return.

All the brothers and sisters are adding in their wishes, dreams, and visions, some of their creation. Some of what they wanted to create, and ran out of time, or were, in some way, prevented from creating. They are posting their desires through you, and letting you know they will be there, empowering you, sending you energy and love throughout your life. You are breathing in all their good intentions, all of their love, blessings, and empowerment.

As you turn, you can feel the Lady. She's almost behind you, yet, she's in you. She's bigger, taller, yet you're inside her, as you walk effortlessly out from that sacred birthing pool. Arriving out, stepping up, stretching, preparing to walk back, feeling strong, full, and boosted; feeling what you're carrying, knowing it's going to come through in the next while; feeling yourself walking with your head held high.

"I'm strong. I'm held in the arms of the Lady of the Lake. I'm safe. I'm well. I am love, and I am loved. And I walk with all of my beloveds who are with me on the inner plane."

As you start walking, you can feel them in your field. They're creating links with you, so they can always return, always come to your call, always be in there in many ways when you call.

Now you're walking back down through the woodlands, down toward the shore. Giving thanks to all of the creatures who have walked with you. Feeling their beautiful kindness, compassion. Walking back, until you can see the shore, the beach, and the barge waiting. Embracing all of the brothers and sisters. All of your beloveds. Feeling you are bigger, stronger, and whole with this part of you that has returned. The Lady beckons you toward the barge, helps you in while you feel her energy and willingness. It's as though you, the Lady, and even the barge, are one energy that she propels forward.

"My beloved, remember I am always here. I never leave your side. I am holding you. You're safe." And as the barge moves off, you can see your brothers and sisters waving; some are crying at your leaving, yet smiling also, knowing only that they love you.

"I'll be back."

You feel yourself turning toward the other shore you can see far in the distance. As you ride out into the center of the lake, you feel this enormous sense of freedom, of release. That old journey is really over.

You speak to the Lady: "My new journey has begun on the inner plane. I have renewed strength within to meet the next part of my journey, the next part of my healing. I can feel the vastness of the burden that has been taken from me. That has been removed from my body, from my bloodline. I give thanks."

The Lady says to you, "That which I have taught you, you will teach others. Yet I will always be leading you from within. I will always be teaching you more. Do not be afraid, my child."

Indeed, the Lady of the Lake within you is a growing fearlessness. As she brings you to the other shore, part of you wants to stay with her and journey forever on her lake, just being with her. As you look out onto the Earth plane, you remember why you came—how much you are needed here, and what you are preparing for. It's almost like getting into gear; you hear the gear click in. You realize how very important it is that you come back fully, and that you bring this love and deep knowing of the Lady into the hearts, minds, and bodies of people.

As you walk back to this moment, feel how strong the presence is. Feel yourself determining never to lose that connection. As if you're making your vows now. The vows that you are preparing to make in the physical realm when you take your priestess vows in Glastonbury. Feel how they are already a reality, that they have been made in many lifetimes. Feel the strength that comes with these vows. You are working your way back to our physical location, right here, in this moment. Back to where your body is. Take your time breathing yourself back in. This new part of you has to get used to this new body, to feeling her. Like when you put a hand in a glove. feel her fully arrive in this body, and feel any emotion that comes up as you return.

"I sense my body feels small to her," I say. "I can feel how long it's been since she's been in a body, and I sense a feeling of amazement at being here. Yet, I also feel she's experiencing some shock, like, 'Wow, we're here. It's time. I'm here now.'"

Give her space to process anything she might need to process.

"She's showing me herself as bloody. I am seeing an image of her in bloody rags."

Yes, yes, she needs to process that; let some of the emotions come.

"It's scary. She doesn't want to be separated again or to be bloody."

Tell her it won't be happening again, but also that you're here for her healing, just as she is here for yours. And that you're remembering, too. Thank her for the memories. Tell her to bring you more. That by bringing them, you're clearing them, together.

"She's showing me some kind of encampment. As though she was outdoors with a group of other priests and priestesses. They were infiltrated, and it was very violent. And fast. Very unexpected. The whole group was killed. Now, I understand so much of what I felt with the group, and the vision, and the journey. She also feels a sense of responsibility as though she's coming back on behalf of the group. They're all coming back through her."

Yes, she's the vessel for healing the whole group. She's done a lot of work on the inner plane, but only soul retrieval can give her the chance to link back to the physical, and get clear. Back to where you have carried this trauma in your body, where this has also been manifesting.

"It feels as though she was stabbed right in the heart."

Breathe into that space. Feel yourself embracing her.

In an instant, I received profound insight and blurted out to Chung Fu, "She was stabbed right where I had the tumor, where the lump appeared."

Right where you had the tumor...Feel the essence and beauty of who she was before this happened. You are drawing her back to herself, all her essence, all her life force, all her beauty. Her soul power. As though you could just step over the devastation and betrayal. The death. The pain of watching those she loved, like parts of herself, being killed.

See yourself reaching out to her as though you are reaching out to someone who is walking forward from the past, which is also your past. Her pure soul that is coming from the spirit world back to you and returns to you also from these memories that enable her, the one who is inside you, to understand her eternal life. Help her let go of the injustice, betrayal, and cruelty. The heartlessness. The mindlessness. Step in and feel her making this choice.

Sometimes when you are feeling her feelings, it helps to find a place in nature where you can sit and just remember. Remember the ones who were taken also walked these lands. Remember their bodies are inside the earth. Honor them with a prayer song and offerings unto the earth. Welcome them home. Welcome them to look through your eyes and remember the beauty of the land. Remember their eternal being is still here, in the land, as part of the land. In the trees and the flowers. Feel their souls journeying with you, on the inner plane. Give thanks for their lives and all they brought and still bring.

How does she—you—feel, now? How are you?

"I can feel how grateful she is that all her brothers and sisters can work through her now."

Excellent. You've been engaged in so many layers of healing.

"So, having the cancer and the tumor is what allowed me to bring her back in?"

Yes.

I sat quietly, just taking in this revelation. Letting it fall inside me. Processing it.

The situation with your mother is also what brought a very big layer of you back in. Because as you realize, this is a massive human drama that has been going on for thousands of years. The alignment of the divine plan, really. The goddess, the creation, that has been going on and on and on. Some of these violent scenarios are layers of the story. There are stories and stories. Some of them have absolutely blocked you. In this life, you have a living story, a "black and white" story, if you will. In it, you literally were closed down, shut down.

Sadly, part of your story is about emotional abuse in the name of kindness, in the name of goodness.

"And in the name of education," I add.

Yes, in the name of doing the right thing through discipline. All in the name of patriarchy, to be honest.

"Exactly." So much was coming together for me at once. I could see that my parents were well-intentioned in their wish for me to have a good education but not aware of the harmful consequences that their decisions would bring to me. They had seen me through the programming of their own lives and experiences; they had both been sent away to boarding school, my father at the tender age of eight. They repeated this pattern with me, without questioning if it really was right for me as an individual.

The school that expelled and medicated me was operating within a patriarchal system that disciplined me for being different, and my parents trusted them as the authority. I know my parents did the best they could at the time. Ultimately, it all unfolded perfectly for me to experience the healing I am now, in this moment. On a soul level, all of this was written in a sacred contract before I was born. My parents and I cocreated the circumstances I needed to bring forward these aspects of myself to be reclaimed.

Yes, you are moving through so many layers. You've become resilient now, strengthened. Strength is your compass now.

My soul family on the inner planes of Avalon had come to my rescue. I had lain facing death in the underworld, in the depths of the unknown, and was gifted the healing water of life to restore me. After being bathed in these holy waters, I was able to reclaim a piece of my soul, a part of me who had been a priestess in Avalon in another time and, because of the fragmentation that occurs during trauma, had not felt safe to move on from that time.

Chung Fu told me when we first started working together that we all have groupings of lifetimes focused on particular themes. We may have several lifetimes focused on learning about forgiveness or compassion, or several lifetimes as a warrior or a teacher, for example. My group of priestess lives were the ones I had come to heal in this lifetime. My soul's intention has been to heal all of the wounds accrued during the grouping of priestess lives, which held a lot of pain, persecution, violence, and suppression.

As I lay naked in the underworld, suspended in time between life and death, I was able to see the deaths of those priestesses I had been. The fragments of those aspects of myself were there, within reach, calling out for me to go to them, to see them, to feel their pain and in so doing, liberate us from it, to unbind the suffering from their power, allowing the purity of their energy to flow back through the waters of life into the blood in my veins, pulsing with new life and possibility.

INANNA'S ASCENT

Gate 7: Retrieval of Her Robe: Choosing Life

Inanna has hung naked on a hook in the underworld for three days and three nights. During this time, she has been initiated into the mysteries of death, where she lets go fully into the realm of the underworld of her dark sister, Ereshkigal. As Inanna hangs on the hook, Ereshkigal moans and cries, unleashing all her pain and anguish. Ereshkigal gives voice to the disowned, lost, fragmented pieces of Inanna that she had not been able to see from her upper-world perspective. In the underworld, Ereshkigal witnesses Inanna's pain, watches her surrender to it, allowing it to move through her body. Inanna allows herself to feel all of it. When her faithful servant comes searching for her in the underworld, Ereshkigal grants her permission to go to Inanna. She feeds her the water of life that will restore her. As Inanna is removed from the hook and reawakens to life, she is told that "no one ascends from the underworld unmarked." If she is to depart and return to her reign in heaven, she must send a sacrifice to take her place. Inanna makes this promise and sets out once more to walk through the seventh gate where she retrieves her robe. The robe is like a healing balm, a layer of comfort and protection over the wounds incurred through violence.

Inanna and I both pull all of our soul energy back in as we walk out of the seventh gate, reclaiming the bodies we have been given and the potent life energy that is here to inhabit them. At the gate of the root chakra, the energy center that governs safety and security, the robe reminds us that we have survived. Neither of us are leaving the underworld the same person we were when we were stripped of that robe. We have faced death, and felt and expressed our pain and despair. In doing so, we retrieved aspects of ourselves that had been lost for time immeasurable. We have been liberated into the knowing of who we truly are. As I slip the robe over my naked body, I sense my system recalibrating to assimilate the influx of energy from my newly reborn priestess self within. Grateful to feel the protective covering of the robe, I bring my arms in close, holding myself. Glancing down toward my heart, I notice the robe is also different. It, too, has been changed in the underworld. It now bears the symbol of the ouroboros: a snake in the shape of a figure eight, eating its own tail. The sight sends a shiver down my spine. Our retrieval has been honored with the symbol of infinity, wholeness, and eternal renewal.

INTEGRATION: WISDOM FROM THE LADY OF THE LAKE

Tune into the elements, your primal self. Enjoy baths, being in the water, burning incense, fire, lighting candles, being outside, and feeling the sunshine. Feel the breeze, listen to the birds, connect with the energy of nature and the elements. Don't look at your phone, computer, or social media. Allow yourself to sink deeper into a healing state. Watching movies is okay; however, social media and the energy of subliminally comparing yourself to others and thinking about what you're going to do after this is over is not supportive. It's not what your brain needs. This (connecting with the elements) will support you in making the most of now as it will plug you into your deepest healer and ancient self.

Through being attuned to that deep primal self, the basic self will be nourished from that line of energy. Healing and insights will surface. Journal and record what arises in whatever way is easiest. You'll be in the healing current that will set the stage for what you can bring through; the state you need to be in for things to come through. There will be plenty of time for mental engagement the rest of your life. This is an opportunity to reside in a deeper space that you need right now.

Bring your mom into your daily meditations in the lake. See her being cleansed of anything that is unlike truth or love, creating the relationship with her you have always desired.

I spoke to Alisha about how I experienced the Lady of the Lake as much more than an archetypal energy. She is a goddess in her own right, a personal guide, an ancient part of me, and yet distinct from my own soul. *What does this mean?*

Alisha explained that my ego was playing into false humility to keep me experiencing myself as separate from Goddess, or in duality consciousness—"*Oh no, I can't be God/Goddess. I can't be Divine.*" The truth is, I *am* Goddess, and everyone else is, too. Yes, that feels big, and it's also ordinary. I am one with all that is. As more was revealed about the journey of my soul and all that I had experienced across the span of my soul's incarnations, I knew this to be true. I was one with it all.

Alisha shared that a necessary element of transformation depends on being honest with what *is* rather than doing a spiritual bypass. Spiritually bypassing refers to the denial of unresolved wounds in an effort to jump too quickly to the spiritual truths we have faith we are but that we have not fully experienced ourselves as yet. We must acknowledge and have empathy for what's present—confusion, doubt, sadness, whatever it is. And then we work to heal and transform these feelings so we ascend the ladder of higher consciousness. We worked with a big karmic piece of self-doubt, an old pattern of me going against myself rather than opening up to my strength.

I forgive myself for judging myself as going against myself.

I forgive myself for judging myself as shutting down rather than challenging another.

I forgive myself for judging myself for avoiding confrontation.

I forgive myself for judging myself as afraid.

I forgive myself for buying into the misbelief that others know best or more than I do.

JOURNAL ENTRY

This morning I experienced full-body shivers for several minutes during meditation as I felt myself bathe in the lake then put on the deep blue robe and crown in the shape of a crescent moon. I felt a deep cellular awakening and integration. I am the Lady of the Lake. The moon crown is a symbol of the wisdom of the celestial realms pouring in. I am a vessel for the Divine, for higher wisdom; starlight shines through my light body. I cycle with the moon, and my bare feet walk the earth, connected to our Great Mother's body, her creatures, her healing energy, her trees, and all of life on this planet. I am a vessel, a channel.

My robe honors my sacred body, and my crown is symbolic and used for attunement to higher information.

Blessed be.

JOURNAL PROMPT

What "cave" within yourself have you feared to enter? What do you feel it contains? What hidden power might you discover there?

MEDITATION

Sit comfortably with your spine straight, or lie down, where you will not be disturbed. Close your eyes, and begin taking in deep diaphragmatic breaths, in through the nose, filling and expanding the belly, and out through the mouth with an audible exhale...ahhh. Repeat three times.

Invite your awareness to focus internally, softening into the darkness within. Begin to visualize your internal landscape as a cave. Scan your body with the intention of observing this terrain. Where are there rocks in the cave? Are there places within you that feel hard or stuck? Areas that hold pain or fear? Where are these places in your body? Is there an area that you instinctively avoid?

Take some time to explore this cave, noticing any feelings that arise.

Choose a particular feeling or sensation and locate where this lives in your body.

Place your hands there and breathe deeply.

Invite the energy that has been stored here to speak, emote, shake, moan, or release in whatever way feels natural.

When you are ready, visualize Inanna with a beautiful vessel of water, here to cleanse this place within you. Feel the purifying energy of the water bringing healing, renewal, and forgiveness.

Once the cleansing is complete, she offers you a beautiful robe. Feel the softness of this sacred garment on your skin as you and Inanna begin your ascent from the underworld, exiting the cave, and walking back across the threshold of the seventh gate.

Slowly come back to the sensation of your hands on your body, observing any shifts that have occurred within your internal landscape.

When you are ready, open your eyes and journal any insights that came forward.

Blessed be.

Chapter Nine

CLAIMING MY DIVINE HERITAGE

SIXTH GATE: PERSONAL AUTHORITY

"When we remember that we are the path and that we must tread it ourselves—lightly, mercifully, consciously—then the healing that goes beyond
'healing' becomes our birthright, and we truly discover ourselves."

~ Stephen Levine

During a spiritual workshop in Los Angeles in 2009, the same year
I became Blue's mom, I was invited to sit in an "Atlantean Healing
Chamber," a pyramid-shaped structure made of copper, crystals, and
fine wood that sat in the living room of the medicine man who was
hosting us. The chamber was one of his own creations. The shift in
the depth of my awareness upon entering this one-person chamber
was immediate. I was overcome with a vision of myself from another
time; I had long, dark, braided hair, and I was walking on green rolling hills wearing woven shoes made of some sort of rope. In the distance, I could see water, and the air around me was misty.

When I emerged, the medicine man smiled and called me "the
Lady of the Lake." It was one of those lightning-bolt moments when

I could feel the truth of his words reverberating through my being. "What does that mean?" I asked. "I'm not sure," he replied. "It just came over me…but in time, you will know."

I was in my first year of school at USM studying spiritual psychology, an interest I had deliberately compartmentalized and kept hidden from most of my friends. I was afraid of being judged and didn't feel safe to share my inner world or anything in the realm of spirituality. I didn't realize at the time that I was in the grips of trauma.

AM I A CHANNEL?

When I was twelve years old, my family moved away from the forests, lakes, and horse pastures of my childhood in Michigan to the small town of Telluride in the Rocky Mountains of Colorado. I started school there in seventh grade. Near the end of that school year, at the age of thirteen, I had a life-defining experience. I was at the town library looking for inspiration for a book report when a woman sitting cross-legged on the floor motioned for me to come over. She asked what I was looking for and suggested casually, "Why don't you write your report about channeling?" I asked her what that was, and she handed me the book *Opening to Channel* by Sanaya Roman and Duane Packer. She said she felt that I was a channel, and that if I wanted to know more about it, to come to her house the next day after school.

In such a small town, only eight blocks long and nestled in a box canyon protected by mountains on three sides, it was common for kids to walk around freely and hang out at various locations before their parents picked them up. I walked to her house excitedly after school, having no idea what I was in for. She invited me to sit in a chair across from her, and I watched her sit silently in meditation. After a short while, her energy shifted, as though another form was coming over her. Her body trembled and moved slightly, then she came back into stillness.

I felt a strong and powerful presence before me and a deep voice came through her. He introduced himself as a Native American spirit guide, and he shared beautiful and accessible wisdom. He reassured me not to fear going against any of the religious beliefs I may have grown up with, that my spiritual path would always lead me to the right place, and that there is no "against-ness" in the world of Spirit. I was in absolute awe and never wanted this encounter to end. I began visiting my new friend regularly and receiving channeling sessions and past-life regressions from her.

Although I didn't comprehend the complexity of this at the time, these experiences awakened my own soul memories of these gifts, and soon, I began channeling one of my spirit guides. I would lie down between the bookshelves in the library of our small-town school and channel for my friends. Throughout eighth grade, this was a regular occurrence. I also began intuitively hypnotizing people. I remember surrounding them in colors, cleansing their auras with incense, and guiding them to breathe into different parts of their bodies and then visualize descending down a flight of stairs. No one taught me this; these abilities felt like deep memories surfacing.

When I was twelve years old, I bought a book from Between the Covers, our local bookshop in Telluride, entitled *Encyclopedia of Ancient and Forbidden Knowledge* by Zolar. On the cover was an image of Stonehenge shimmering in the light of a full moon. This was around the same time I met the woman who inspired my first opening as a channel. I don't remember anything I read in that book, but the image of Stonehenge burned in my brain. I slept with the book right next to me on my bedside table, staring into the image of the stones.

At age sixteen, I traveled to England, Ireland, and Scotland with my family, and vividly remember feeling overcome with a sense of being home in Scotland near Loch Ness. I loved experiencing different parts of the world, and by the time I was thirty, I had spent a significant amount of time traveling with the aim of spiritual exploration. I spent time in ashrams in India, visited sacred sites in Sri Lanka, immersed myself in silent meditation at a Buddhist Monastery in Thailand, made offerings in the beautiful temples of Bali, discovered the spiritual nature of tea in Taiwan, drank tea with tea masters in remote and exquisitely beautiful parts of China, and sat with shamans for plant medicine ceremonies in Peru.

I woke up on New Year's Day, at thirty-two, filled with longing to return to England on a pilgrimage, to visit the stones and walk the sacred landscape I knew was such a deep part of me. I booked my trip that morning, and the following summer went on a life-changing pilgrimage led by Mara Freeman. My first night sleeping in the retreat center, I woke to a presence in my room. As my eyes adjusted in the dark, I saw and felt clearly a woman with dark hair, wearing a long maroon-colored skirt with a dagger fastened around her waist. I knew she was Morgan Le Fey. She reached out her hand and said, *"Come with me..."* and instantly I was swept away into an ecstatic vision, flying with her over the land, looking down at stone circles, sacred mounds, rivers, wells, and streams. She looked at me—we were both glimmering with starlight, her aura illuminated by the moon—and said, *"Welcome home, sister."* The next thing I knew I was sitting back in my bed in the retreat center, bleary eyed and buzzing with excitement.

I completely fell in love with Glastonbury and never wanted to leave, a feeling that has remained with me since. Glastonbury is known as "the land of shimmering crossroads." There are many ways to experience this wondrous place. Some simply enjoy the outer beauty of the landscape and the interesting shops on the High Street, while others are drawn through gateways into the spirit realm, where they may encounter the ancient and mystical power of the sacred land of Avalon. I heard a wise elder once say that if Avalon takes you as her own, you will never really leave. I welled up with tears when I heard these words, as this has been my experience. My life changed when I stepped foot on those lands and the Goddess claimed me as Her priestess. After that first journey to Avalon, it was clear I could no longer deny the full truth of who I am. I longed to connect with my true lineage of magic, to know my divine heritage, to honor the path I had come here to remember.

WITCH CAMP

In the years leading up to training as a Priestess of Avalon, I was involved with the Reclaiming community, a movement created and cofounded by Starhawk. I took classes in the back of a magical shop in North Hollywood, learning about casting circles and working with the elements, creating potions for active dreaming, and strengthening my will. For a couple years, I took every class I could, attended a witch camp in the redwoods of Northern California, and went through a yearlong priestess training in sacred leadership.

Many gifts came from my time with Reclaiming. I obviously have always connected with being a witch. Being in a safe space that honored this spiritual path was deeply comforting to my inner teenager. I remember at the time being so fragmented and afraid that I would never tell anyone what I was doing. I would say I was going on a camping trip with friends; never would I have dared to say the words "witch camp."

It was the same with spiritual psychology. I told friends I was taking psychology classes, not that I was immersed in a two-year experiential master's program in spiritual psychology. I was so afraid of the backlash, shame, and punishment that I had experienced as a teenager that I refused to create any kind of opening into my inner world, except with the few special friends who were sharing these experiences with me. Yet, I noticed how carefree they all were about sharing what they were doing—"*Mom, I'm going to witch camp!*"—and posting a photo in their cape on Facebook. That terrified me, and I would literally tell them that wasn't safe and to please stop. I have so much compassion for myself now that I understand the depth of the pain and fragmentation I was walking with.

Opening the doorway to remembering the witch within started my path of honoring the truth of my heart. After the boarding school incident, I felt that what my heart longed for was somehow bad or wrong. I began to fear the longing in me to work with magic—spells, herbs, potions, and candles. I was afraid that the deep desires of my heart were forbidden. I noticed that anything associated with witchcraft, magic, or the Goddess was demeaned as "less than" and not appropriate or acceptable by patriarchal culture, and I worried that made me "less than." I felt I was less than those who practiced modern religion or other forms of new-age mysticism, and these judgments weighed heavily on me. I was so painfully afraid of being seen as bad or wrong.

When I had the courage to embark on my spiritual path as an adult at age twenty-six, I found myself in situations where Christian-based language was used. For example, prayers beginning with, *"Lord God of all creation," "Our Father, who art in heaven,"* or *"In the name of the Father."* There was a part of me that believed this type of language was right and superior, and that the deep stirrings within me to honor the earth, the elements, and the Goddess would be seen as wrong and inferior in the eyes of those around me.

I had a deep longing for a spiritual framework to my life, so I continued to follow the path as it unfolded, slowly learning to identify the internal patriarchal programming that was preventing me from accepting myself. I remember crying to a friend about how I was yearning to follow the path of the priestess, but that I felt such a strong inner conflict about that path being wrong.

"Why can't I just choose something more socially acceptable, like studying A Course in Miracles?" I had asked. The truth is, to be a witch or a priestess is not a choice; it is a *sacred calling.* My choice was either to listen to the whisperings of my heart, knowing this was

guidance from my soul pointing me toward my truth, or live a life of denial bound up in the suppression of outdated thought forms and the opinions of others.

When I got cancer, I realized that this was literally a life-or-death choice for me. I could not go through one more lifetime denying the truth of who I am. Working with Alisha brought me face-to-face with the fear of my path being "less than" anything constructed with biblical or Christian language. She herself used Christian and esoteric language, yet she was inspired to embrace and honor the Goddess through me. She told me simply that she had been working with the language she had learned, but it was exciting to be exposed to Spirit through the goddesses I experienced. She immediately changed her prayers and language to include the goddesses I worked with, and told me that including the goddesses had expanded her experience of how the essence of Spirit (Source consciousness) communicates—through exquisitely beautiful forms that reach people in the way they can best receive Spirit/Source. She was able to start tuning into the goddesses with me to allow them to assist my healing. Even though she felt she hadn't consciously known the goddesses in this lifetime, she was able to attune to and love them through our shared intention of my healing and connecting to the Divine.

We talked about the distinction between the path of witchcraft and the path of the priestess. A witch uses her will to cocreate magic with the elements and, in her highest expression, experiences oneness with the elements and, therefore, the Divine. A priestess surrenders her will to Divine will, allowing the magic of Goddess and the elements to flow through her.

During times of experiencing physical pain and suffering during treatment, Alisha created simple exercises to help me come back to a place of truth within. First, I would acknowledge what *is*. *What was I feeling? What was I thinking?* I would check in to see how my little girl inside was doing and be honest with myself about what I really wanted at that moment. Second, I would go to Spirit and ask, "What's good about this?"

Some common answers I received are:

This is how my Sight opens up after twenty-two years.

This is how I heal maternal karma.

This is how I model spiritual transformational healing.

This is part of the spiritual transformation and not separate from it.

I am learning to reside in the knowing that what is mine cannot be taken from me.

This is how I claim my divine heritage.

MY FIRST PRIESTESS SELF

At Samhain, in November, I sat on the slopes of the Tor with my priestess group and our teacher, Luna. It had been only days since Blue's passing, and my heart was heavy with grief. I carried a persistent aching lump in my breast that had just appeared on the plane ride over. It was the first weekend of our second spiral, and we had been out walking the land. We settled into the apple orchard, on the south side of the ancient isle, and Luna guided us in a mediation to meet our first priestess self, the first priestess incarnation our souls had experienced.

I am walking through a lush green jasmine-scented pathway. Blue picks me up on his back, and I see that he has Pegasus wings. We fly through time, through dimensions and wormholes, and come out at a very ancient sandstone cave with a low entrance. I walk into the cave and fall down a tunnel...

There is a beautiful round ancient doorway in the earth; I crawl through and cross a threshold into a magical open space with high

ceilings and an amazing amount of light, considering I am under-
ground. There are paintings all over the cave. A woman wearing
animal skins, bone jewelry, and furs stands before me. She has big
brown eyes. She begins dancing around and painting herself with
blood, painting spirals and symbols on her body and mine. She speaks
about blood as a medium to the sacred, to the source of life, to carry
me between the worlds. She tells me that a priestess creates space for
communication between the worlds.

I see my old home, burrowed in the side of the Tor. There is a fire and
hanging herbs; I feel water and mist all around me. There are stand-
ing stones nearby, covered in thick green moss, and an old well. In my
home, a cave dwelling within the hillside, the water flows within the
earth. There is a pool of water, surrounded by stone, and I gaze into
it. In a loud and clear voice, I hear the question, "Who are you?" In
almost deafening waves reverberating through my being, a reply comes
forth: "I am the Lady of the Lake, I am the Lady of the Lake" over
and over again.

I felt shy about sharing this with my group when Luna asked. My
small mind was in disbelief and saying things like, "Who do you
think you are to claim something like that?"

I hesitantly shared when asked, and was open about the embar-
rassment I felt. Luna's words soothed my heart as she reminded me
how important it is to trust what comes through when we are accessing the deep wisdom and memory of our souls, and that our human
selves are programmed to do the opposite. We are programmed to
think critically and, emotionally, to play small. The mind says, "Who
are you to do that?" We spoke more about it later, and I expressed
my desire to learn more about the Lady of the Lake. I asked for
book recommendations, as I'd never seen much written about her.
Luna smiled, her eyes brimming with mystery, and she said, "That's
because it's yours to write."

JOURNAL ENTRY, MESSAGE FROM THE LADY OF THE LAKE

I am here. I have returned. I bring with me ancient and forgotten wisdom of our sisterhood, our healing ways and knowledge. I have come to bring this through in service to the healing and awakening of the old ways of being. This will create a vibratory shift on the planet that will tip the scales in the direction of higher consciousness, loving, and remembering. The memories that have unlocked have also been unlocked in your sisters. Working together is a key to the discovery of these memories. The transmissions are there in your hands and will come through in the resonance of the group field.

INANNA'S ASCENT

Gate 6: Retrieval of the Lapis Measuring Rod: Personal Authority

As Inanna ascends through the sixth gate of the underworld, she retrieves her lapis measuring rod. This gate is connected with the sacral chakra, below the navel, which governs her relationships and the way she uses her primal feminine energy. As she takes the lapis rod into her hand, she recognizes that although this can be used as a tool for measuring the truth of souls, her deepest sense of truth resides within her. She can use things outside of her as resources for discernment; however, she is now her own personal authority, a power that exists beyond what can be contained in any object. As she begins to collect the trappings of her life in the upper world, she no longer identifies with them. They are not what make her queen. The royalty of her being comes from the heritage of her soul. She takes confident steps, feeling liberated by her experience in the underworld.

WHAT'S FOR YOU WON'T GO BY YOU

"What's for you won't go by you" is a saying I heard in Scotland in the summer of 2017 in the time leading up to my first priestess dedication, just before I was diagnosed. This saying echoed through me as I communed with the wild land of Scotland. I felt comforted in knowing that what was truly for me, for my highest good, would not pass me by. Strands of the woven basket of my spiritual heritage were coming together, offering me threads of remembering. I recognized that as long as I am clear inside and my intentions are pure, the best I can do is follow the yearnings of my heart. I trust that when I align my will to the will of the Divine, asking for the highest good of all concerned to be brought forward, my aim will always be true.

The only time I doubted or second-guessed my magic or my true desires was when I compared myself to others or overvalued others' perceptions of me. What's for them is *for them*, and what's for me is *for me*. To compare my path to someone else's spiritual curriculum and the material they have come here to work through is to completely miss the point. I am here to reclaim the magical woman within, and ultimately, that has nothing to do with anyone else. It is between Goddess and me.

PRIESTESS OF AVALON

Dedicating as a Priestess of Avalon in July of 2019 as a breast cancer survivor was a glorious experience:

During my ceremony, I feel the presence of my ancient community in Avalon by my side. I feel my young priestess self, integrated within me, free to express herself and her magic.

I am walking through an ancient temple, through dark passageways lit by torches, surrounded by columns of light, my feet touching earth and stone.

Further into the darkness I walk, held by the spiritual energies that support me, toward the heart of the Lady of Avalon.

As I sit before Her, my mind is empty; I have no thoughts. My consciousness expands out beyond the ceremonial space, past the boundaries of the sacred landscape, up into the night sky, where I eventually merge with a star. I feel my original existence as a twinkling star, one with all that is. I am overcome with a profound sense of peace, shining as a star, part of the magnificent tapestry of the universe.

I am one with the Source of all.

As I ascend through the sixth gate of the underworld, I am sovereign.

JOURNAL ENTRY, MESSAGE FROM MY YOUNG PRIESTESS SELF

Indeed, I am very old; however, you may call me your young priestess self. Feel us together in Avalon, filled, surrounded, held within the all-encompassing loving, healing embrace of Goddess. We are one now. You are healing and coming through transformed and renewed. You have found the treasure. Allow yourself to relax and honor what feels right in each moment. I love you dearly. Your mother is healing too, and that healing energy is rippling out through your feminine lineage. Release your fears about others and trust they, too, are held in divine love and protection. Blessed be.

JOURNAL PROMPT

How would it feel to be powerful beyond measure? To know that you are one with the infinite Source of all creation? Who would you be if this were true?

MEDITATION

Sit comfortably with your spine straight, or lie down, where you will not be disturbed. Close your eyes, and begin taking in deep diaphragmatic breaths, in through the nose, filling and expanding the belly, and out through the mouth with an audible exhale...ahhh. Repeat three times.

Placing your hands over your low belly, ask inside to connect to the eternal wisdom and power of your soul. You are a multidimensional being, human and divine all at the same time, and your potential is vast. Visualize a shimmering crystal reflecting prisms of light in different directions. These different rays of light and their kaleidoscope of color represent your soul's unique design and blueprint. Similar to the geometry of a snowflake, no two are alike. As you bask in the brilliance of your inner light, your awareness expands into the understanding that these rays are offering a pathway, guiding you to your divine Self. Allow yourself to breathe and meditate here, experiencing the power of your own divine presence, the part of you who knows that you are one with the infinite Source of all creation.

This aspect of you understands your unique purpose on this earth and reminds you that playing small is not in service to its fulfillment.

You feel a question arising from deep within: "Who would I be if I allowed myself to expand into the vastness of my divine potential?"

Allow your mind to soften, letting go of any expectations, while remaining open to whatever comes forward.

When you have received a feeling, an insight, an image, or a direct knowing, feel that frequency pulsing out from your center and filling your body with light. Feel a sense of reclamation of the truth of who you are as a divine being having a human experience.

See Inanna standing before you, her lapis rod in her hand. She reminds you that you are your own authority, that no one understands the deep wisdom and magic of your soul more profoundly than you do. Standing anchored in the truth of this knowing, together you walk across the threshold of the sixth gate of the underworld.

Breathe deeply while feeling your hands on your body, offering gratitude for the eternal wisdom that resides within you.

When you are ready, open your eyes and journal any insights that came forward.

Blessed be.

Chapter Ten

TRANSFORMATION CEREMONY

FIFTH GATE: EMBODYING MY POWER

"Insights from myth, dreams, and intuitions, from glimpses of an invisible reality, and from perennial human wisdom provide us with hints and guesses about the meaning of life and what we are here for."

~ Jean Shinoda Bolen

I'M (NOT) IN SPONTANEOUS REMISSION

When I first started treatment, I "decided" that I would experience a miraculous healing while going through chemo and not need any kind of surgery. This was my prayer. As I progressed into the medical experience, I made agreements with myself that allowed me to stay present with what was happening right in front of me and not dissociate due to the immense shock and trauma of it all. *It was easier for me to accept chemo if I told myself I wouldn't need surgery.*

My life had been on a certain trajectory before cancer, at least in my mind. I had been married for two and a half years, and my husband

and I were ready to have kids. I fantasized about being pregnant and giving birth. I envisioned traveling to Glastonbury with a full belly, life growing in my womb—perhaps a reincarnated priestess sister was coming to be with me again. I dreamed of names and carried lists of girl and boy names on my phone. I imagined a home birth with the primal sound of drums filling the space while I writhed and moaned in the blessed ecstasy of childbirth. I looked forward to knowing what it felt like to give birth. I'd had the honor of attending several births as a doula (a nonmedical birthing assistant) and was deeply moved witnessing the process. I always thought, *I can't wait to feel that in my body*. I have always had a gift for sitting with people in pain, unapologetically meeting them where they are and holding them in loving care and regard. No one wants to feel pitied, especially in our most vulnerable moments. These tender places are where we are closest to Spirit. When the veils of socially acceptable behavior and the masks of being "put together" for the outside world fall away, we meet the raw, wild, primal, creative force of life within. We connect with our power.

I experienced this not by giving birth to a baby but by having a mastectomy.

TERAPHIM AND TSELEM

From February to the beginning of April, while I was existing deep in the underworld enduring the light infusion treatments, I chanted to myself daily, "I am in spontaneous remission! I am saving my left breast!" When I let myself think about the possibility of having my left breast removed, it felt as if my heart was crumbling; the pain was insurmountable. My prayer circle sisters supported me in my vision of saving my left breast, and that goal as a focal point helped me have a purpose in my daily meditations. I was eradicating the cancer and saving my breast.

During this time, I went to see two beautiful healers, who work together as embodiments of the Divine Mother and Divine Father, Tselem and Teraphim. I met Tselem one auspicious day in Glastonbury. I was enjoying an hour of free time in the middle of a retreat I was leading and decided to stop on the High Street for my favorite turmeric hot chocolate. A woman standing barefoot in priestess robes was at the counter placing her order. She seemed beyond the bounds of time; she could have, and maybe *had*, walked through an ancient portal and right into this café. Now, it's common to see all kinds of people in any kind of outfit you can imagine in Glastonbury, but this woman was different. As I stood near her, I felt my entire energy field shift. We began to speak and everything around me dropped away—my vision blurred until I was standing in a big golden orb and all I could see within it were her eyes. This encounter had a big impact on me that I felt for weeks. I went back to the retreat center and told my friend Ashley I had just met an ascended master in human form. Several months later when I was going through the light infusions, one of my prayer circle sisters sent me a meditation from two healers she was working with—a man and woman, who transmitted Divine Mother and Divine Father energies. There was a photo at the bottom of the email, and to my amazement, it was the woman from the café in Glastonbury. They were in San Diego; Ryan drove me down to see them. I had an incredibly potent session with them. The powerful force of Goddess palpably moved through Tselem like thunder as she commanded specific karmic wounds and imprints to be released from my soul. I felt myself residing in a space of oneness with all creation. As I sat across from them with my eyes closed, I felt myself in a tornado of energy, releasing, shifting, recoding. At the end of the session, I asked about my breast. They responded that the most important thing was that I make the choice deeply from within, from my own Sovereignty. *That's what this whole journey is about.*

MRI: THERE'S NOTHING THERE

When I went for an MRI at the end of April, I felt supercharged and ready to see the culmination of all the spiritual healing in physical-world reality—in my body. While lying in the MRI machine, I had a vision of the Lady of the Lake.

She is walking before me in her sapphire blue robes, guiding me up a winding path of green moss and stone to a hot spring pool. I am delighted to soak in these healing waters. The air is crisp and fresh, and my body is relaxed. We plunge underwater and swim into a tunnel that leads up into another pool. Here, the water is warm, and there is a cold waterfall nearby. We walk to her cave dwelling and warm ourselves by the fire, sipping fresh spring water. I lay down by the fire to receive her healing; she is moving symbols of waving lines through my energy field. A group of priestess students are accompanying her.

The results of the MRI were crystal clear—a miracle truly had occurred. I immediately sent the results to my prayer circle, highlighting the words *no masses or enhancement are demonstrated; the appearance is compatible with complete response to neoadjuvant chemotherapy. The study demonstrates no MRI evidence of malignancy.*

"*There's nothing there!!!*" I exclaimed. I was over the moon and felt my prayer of saving my breast had been answered. My prayer circle sisters rejoiced, and we all cried happy tears while exchanging excited messages of victory. Shortly after, a text came through from my surgeon:

MRI is not microscopic pathology. You could easily harbor residual cancer cells in multiple locations that want to make a debut back again someday soon. The MRI DOES NOT RESOLVE LESS THAN a 5mm wad of cancer. Mastectomy is still your best option. I would not change my mind based on the MRI. But!! Super great news in terms of prognosis that it looks totally clear!

A common feeling during the journey with cancer was having the wind knocked out of me. Moments of elation and success followed by a blow to the stomach. I spoke with my oncologist about the decision, and he sagely and eloquently communicated his message in a way that reminded me of the serenity prayer often spoken in twelve-step programs:

Goddess, grant me the serenity to accept the things I cannot change

The courage to change the things I can

And the wisdom to know the difference.

He encouraged me to accept that I could not change what had already happened, that I had gotten cancer. It helped when I framed this advice within the context of the serenity prayer. This doctor suggested I use my "cosmic powers," as he called them, to change the things I could. By this, he meant continue to do the mind-body-spirit work I had already begun. By now, I had become a master at reframing issues as blessings and finding the silver lining in every situation I was faced with. I enjoyed viewing this as "changing the things I can." This is where the understanding of my cancer experience as a spiritual opportunity and initiation comes in. The "wisdom to know the difference" is about using discernment. There are environmental factors and myriad other things that contribute to dis-ease on the physical level that we cannot control (or can, but only to a certain degree, through lifestyle choices) and don't fully understand. "Living the wisdom" is making the most aligned choices for my health and longevity, while not needing to prove anything to anyone else about spiritual healing.

I DIDN'T SAY YOU WERE CURED

Alisha had told me months prior that her spiritual teacher, John Roger, had said, "Karma is cleared with a knife." When I first heard this statement, I shuddered; it felt so powerful and true. As I was grappling with the impending surgery, diving within to really feel what my body wanted and needed, Alisha told me a story. A woman with breast cancer attended a lecture with John Roger, who would often offer intuitive wisdom to participants. The woman was in a similar position as I—she was scheduled for surgery but hoping and trying to find another way. John Roger said, "A woman with breast cancer has had a great spiritual healing today" to the crowd. "You know who you are; come speak with me after."

Overjoyed, the woman rushed to speak with him. "Does this mean I don't need surgery?" she asked. John Roger replied, "I said you received a spiritual healing; I didn't say you were cured." As I heard this story, I understood with more clarity the complexity of healing. There are so many layers involved, each one intertwined with individual stories, beliefs, ancestral patterns, karmic wounds, and opportunities for healing and awakening in this lifetime. It was just so complex. It slowly began to occur to me that the option most aligned with my spiritual healing might be surgery. If karma is cleared with a knife, perhaps the eradication and removal of this karmic wound depended on its physical extraction. This began to make sense.

A sister from prayer circle sent me a story about Amazon warrior women who cut off one breast as a symbol of their sovereignty. Perhaps this was my true warrioress initiation. All of this was confirmed, without a shadow of a doubt, when my doctors told me my mastectomy surgery was scheduled for June 1, my mother's birthday. After all the work reclaiming my maiden self, healing the unmothered parts of me, and releasing the ancestral pain of my mother line, the mother wound would be physically extracted from my body while in the energetic portal of my mother's birthday.

MESSAGE TO PRAYER CIRCLE

Hi, beautiful prayer circle sisters,

I have some news. I had a long meeting with Dr. Piro yesterday. He reviewed all my records, including scans and every image I have— everything. My intention was to receive his neutral opinion, as my oncologist, about the next steps forward regarding surgery.

During our meeting, it became crystal clear to me, at a deep level, that I am going to be getting a mastectomy. This is my choice, and I'm very clear that's what I need to do, for many reasons. I understand now that if I do nothing and leave the breast tissue in my body, there's a high chance of cancer coming back within the year.

It's just way too risky.

Even when I was contemplating this and thinking about the possibilities leading up to my decision, I was wondering if I would be able to have any sense of peace knowing that all of that tissue was in my body. I really feel this choice will give me the most peace of mind moving forward.

I'm turning thirty-seven on Sunday; I don't want to ever fucking get cancer again.

This has been the most brutal experience. I mean, honestly. I know I have held myself in the most powerful way, and it has been an extraordinary initiation. I have experienced such profound healing, as I have done the deepest work of my life. And, I have also been enduring torture. I mean that it has been so painful. I feel like I've had my head held under water for six months at this point. I never, ever want to fucking go through this again. I'm very clear about this.

When I hear statistics and the absolute, matter-of-fact information coming from Dr. Piro, I know there really isn't even a decision to be made. He's also saying, "I never want you to get this again. This is the way to ensure there won't be any cancer left in your body."

He encouraged me to focus on the good news—that I get to save my nipple, and a lot of women don't. This means they basically pull the skin up, make an incision, and remove all of the tissue. Then insert an implant, and sew my skin back on. I will have a little scar, but my breast will look similar to its natural state from the outside.

Emotionally, this sounds really supportive. This way, I know that the tissue and all of those unhealthy cells are out of me.

Hopefully they won't tell me I have to also do radiation. I really don't want to do that. I feel a stronger "no" about radiation than I did about surgery.

Dr. Piro explained more to me about the MRI technology. Even though it looks clear in the image, on a microscopic, biological level, there can still be residue there that could reproduce, especially with the level of cancer that I had. Mine was a severe grade, advanced, and invasive. It had been in my body for a long time without being detected. There is all kinds of terrifying information about ways the cancer could manifest more extremely if the tissue isn't removed.

This is all I need to know. I feel completely on board and okay with this. This is my path. This is what needs to happen. This is what Spirit and Goddess are putting in front of me.

This is what I'm doing next. I'm calling on the Amazon women who sacrificed one of their breasts as a symbol of their sovereignty. I'm really holding to that vision and accepting that this is part of the alchemical journey for me.

My femininity is not contained in the tissue inside my breast.

I'll still have my right breast.

Having this surgery is the completion of the warrior journey.

I feel like I have all of the support around me that I need, especially from all of you. Please help me hold this experience as a powerful karmic clearing that will result in a substantial shift in consciousness for me.

I feel strongly that this is an action toward life, a life-affirming choice. I want to live a long, healthy life, and be a grandmother. This is what I know I need to do to make that happen. The spirit world has confirmed this for me by scheduling the surgery on my mom's birthday, June 1. So much of my healing has been around the maiden, healing the unmothered parts of me, and my mother line.

Thank you for being the most amazing sisters in the world. I love you all so much.

Blessed be.

SECOND MESSAGE TO PRAYER CIRCLE

Hi, sisters,

It is very important to me that the news/choice I shared with you today is held in sacredness and surrounded with love. Please no sadness or apologies. I've just come from a powerful session with Alisha and feel so clear that this is the deepest level of healing for me and what I desire. She encouraged me not to talk to too many people about my decision and to hold only loving thoughts for my healing. I am asking you to help me hold this sacred container as I move toward this experience on June 1. Thank you!

. . .

REFRAMING MY SURGERY

Alisha helped me to reframe the surgery as my transformation ceremony, and from that moment on, I spoke of it only in that way. I held this decision close to my heart and shared with dear friends who would also hold it sacred and view my surgery as my transformation ceremony. I had no space for people who might want to feel sorry for me. In fact, having people say, "I'm sorry" to me all the time was the worst feeling ever. I never felt better or comforted hearing it. The messages that lifted me up were ones of acknowledgment and encouragement. The ones that acknowledged the fire I was walking through and reminded me what a strong, courageous, and badass woman I am. I loved knowing my friends were with me, rooting for me, and believing in me. When I was going through chemo, I was very private and selective about who I allowed to visit me. I was so raw and emotionally vulnerable, and my physical appearance changed so drastically, that I felt safest only with those who witnessed every stage of my journey. When those close friends came to visit, it was a welcome reprieve from my underworld cave. I had experienced what it felt like for people who hadn't seen me since I'd lost my healthy appearance and my long, shiny blonde hair. When they saw me swollen, red-faced, and bald, it was actually unbearable to experience them seeing me and feeling their shock and sadness. Their tears didn't comfort and console me or remind me of the strong warrioress I am. I felt the same as always on the inside; I was still me. When my close prayer circle sisters who were standing by my side cried with me—and there was a lot of crying—it was a different kind of crying, cathartic and beautiful. I began to understand, with a measure of personal pain, that many people don't know how to respond to someone with a life-threatening illness and serious medical protocols. They can come across as insensitive, afraid, and dismissive.

A few times before I decided to move forward with the transformation ceremony, a couple of friends, on different occasions, tried to console me as I faced the potential loss of my breast by referring to it as "just tissue." I imagine this was an attempt at lightening the magnitude of the decision ahead of me, but it had the opposite effect. These flippant words seriously undermined my feelings and process even though I understood it to be spiritual bypassing: using the spiritual idea of "you are not your body" to avoid deeper, more painful feelings. I realized it was up to me to be compassionate, to be the stronger one, and accept that they simply didn't have the experience and, therefore, sensitivity to behave differently. These experiences taught me to hold the transformation ceremony sacred and private.

I made this choice near the end of April, after my sixth and final round of chemo. On April 29, 2018—my thirty-seventh birthday—I went for a hike with Bonne and Val, two dear prayer circle sisters. I had drawn a vibrant and colorful picture of my left breast, covered in sacred goddess symbols and Avalon imagery, on biodegradable paper. When we reached a plateau overlooking the ocean, I called in the goddesses of the Wheel of Bridannia as we stood beneath an oak tree. My sisters helped me dig a hole, where I symbolically "buried" my left breast. I thanked her for being a part of me for thirty-seven years, for her beauty, for the symbol of femininity, sexuality and nourishment she had been. I thanked her for the loving sacrifice she was making for the healing of my mother line and my soul. I sprinkled drops of water from the Red and White springs in Avalon and added rose petals, chocolate, apple seeds, and a few drops of frankincense into her grave. As I buried her, pushing the soil with my hands, I released all remaining emotions I had about the surgery—and the loss—into the earth.

I decided to go to the Optimum Health Institute in San Diego, which offers a raw-food cleansing and healing program, to detox from chemo and prepare for surgery. During this time, I focused on purging all the physical, mental, and emotional toxins I could. I was fortunate to be with two great friends, one who had been through breast cancer, and we laughed and cried together as we drank green juice and cleansed. It was the first time in months I was able to stomach anything green, and that in itself felt like a huge triumph. It's incredible to experience the emotional memories that arise while physically cleansing. We were walking laps around the periphery of the grounds and telling each other stories from high school, about old boyfriends, and things we hadn't thought of in many years.

I was practicing a daily exercise Alisha had taught me to prepare for my transformation coming up on June 1. I called in the Light, Source, Divine Mother and Father, all the goddesses, my guides, angels, higher Self, and basic self. I called in the Lady of the Lake, Archangel Saamprael (according to Alisha, this is the great archangel who bridges the archangelic and goddess consciousness), Brigid, the Lady of Avalon, Venus, Sekhmet, Mary Magdalene, and the Spirit doctors of Avalon. Envisioning a chalice full of light in front of my heart, I energetically placed all that I was releasing with the surgery into the chalice, letting it all go. I physically gestured with my hands, removing specific fears and old self-defeating patterns from where I experienced them in my body and placing them in the chalice. The unconscious doesn't know the difference between an action taken in everyday reality versus one performed within the context of a ritual, and this is one reason that ritual is such a powerful catalyst for transformation. Once the chalice was full and contained all that had been released, I closed it with my hands. I then lifted the chalice over my head, offering it up to Spirit. *Poof!* I trusted everything would be transmuted. Now I could focus on refilling these spaces within me, with what I needed to move forward, and with the vision of who I wanted to be and how I wanted to feel when I woke up from surgery. I wrote an ideal scene, a skill I'd learned from my spiritual psychology program at USM, about how I would feel after surgery:

> *I am waking up from my transformation ceremony feeling fantastic! I am experiencing bliss, joy, and love. I am experiencing a palpable shift into higher levels of consciousness.*

I am feeling tremendous gratitude, love, and tenderness for my body.

I am thrilled to be completely free and clear of dis-ease! I am experiencing radiant health and vitality beaming from every cell in my body and reverberating through all levels of consciousness.

My body and I are welcoming my left breast in her new form, integrating her with grace, ease, and bliss. She looks and feels gorgeous.

I am grateful my skin has healed so quickly and beautifully. My skin is luminous.

I am loving and trusting my surgeons, nurses, and anesthesiologist. I am feeling held, safe, and protected.

These are just a few of the sentences I recorded myself speaking aloud. As June 1 drew closer, I listened to my ideal scene and visualized releasing my fears into the image of the chalice of light multiple times a day. A few days before the transformation ceremony, I saw my reconstructive surgeon, Dr. Tiffany Grunwald. Because she was the one placing the new energy into my body with the implant, I asked her if she would be willing to read a prayer aloud when this time came during surgery. She was moved by the request and graciously said yes. I had written my prayer on a Brigid card from the Goddess Temple in Glastonbury, which she then took into the operating room (OR) with her on June 1.

During the four hours under anesthesia, I had a nipple-sparing, skin-sparing mastectomy and breast reconstruction. I was very fortunate to be able to save my skin and nipple because this isn't always possible. A few weeks prior, I'd had a shorter surgery in which Dr. Kristi Funk made the mastectomy cut, pulled the skin away, took some of the duct from behind my left nipple to biopsy, and then sewed my skin back. She invented this technique called a nipple-delay. Essentially, it disconnects all the blood vessels that fed the skin from the tissue below, so that the blood vessels create new pathways to keep the skin and nipple alive without being dependent on the tissue that would be removed. Brilliant. My nipple looks alive and responds to touch, rather than being a different color and flat like a pancake.

Over the course of six months, I went under anesthesia three times. The first was on December 24, just after I was diagnosed, for the egg retrieval. When I woke up, I immediately began exclaiming to Ryan, "Goddesses are real! I was in Avalon! Goddesses are real!" I shared with him that I had traveled to Avalon, where a circle of goddesses held me in a sacred ceremony during the procedure. They shared their intention to assist me during this journey of transfiguration by bringing me into direct connection with my ancient self—the part of me who remembers who I am and why I am here. After this experience, I asked Ryan if he would record me when I came out of anesthesia to capture what was coming through me, as I had no recollection of it once I recovered.

My voice is scratchy in the recordings because I had breathing tubes down my throat during both surgeries. While my speech is labored; my words are lucid. It's an interesting juxtaposition to listen to the powerful messages pouring through me with the beeps of machines and hospital noises in the background. I have no conscious memory of anything I said after either procedure. After my nipple-sparing surgery on May 7, these were my words:

I felt the spirit of Sheela Na Gig (an ancient goddess depicted in carvings throughout Europe as an old woman squatting and holding her vulva open); I went through her yonic gateway. I passed through a portal, a passage, of the dark goddess. The Lady of the Lake held my inner maiden and Archangel Saamprael held my inner child, letting them both know they are safe. There was so much protection. I felt a column of light around me, seeping into my skin. I felt myself breathing in the light that was above my head, below my feet, and all around me. I released so much—old baggage and limiting beliefs. I feel a deep clearing and a shift in my consciousness and can see how these surgical procedures are part of the clearing of my journey. I feel such a relief; so much has been lifted and cleared.

I felt Yeshua in the room, and Mary Magdalene, and Brigid, and the Lady of Avalon. I feel so much lightness around my head. All of my gifts have returned to me through this opening. I'm in a place of transformation. I feel my feet on the path of awakening; this is a momentous, far-reaching turning point.

I felt I was in the realms of light; the spirit doctors from Avalon and Chung Fu surrounded me. When I entered the light, I felt that my breast was ready to make this sacrifice for the rest of my life, healing, transformation, and the sanctity and longevity of the rest of my body. I feel now that my gifts will open, that they are open. This is the beginning of my radiant empowered life. I feel so much light around me. So much rainbow light. In every cell of my body. I feel the divine feminine, angelic presence that works through Dr. Funk, and the conduit she is for divine healing and clearing wounds in the collective unconscious of women. She has an angelic presence that I could feel so much on my left side.

A few weeks later, on June 1, my mother's birthday, I arrived at St John's Hospital in Santa Monica in the wee hours of the morning. The mastectomy surgery was an approximately four-hour procedure. The first half was Dr. Funk's removal of my breast and thirteen lymph nodes, and the second half was Dr. Grunwald's reconstruction. For the reconstruction, she used an implant along with stem cell tissue. As Dr. Grunwald read the prayer I had given her, the OR went completely silent. These are the words she spoke as she placed the implant in my body:

I call on Taylor's highest Self, her guides, angels, Mother Goddess and Father God, and all the goddesses who support her.

May this implant be tuned perfectly to the harmony of Taylor's body. May it be filled with divine love, sacredness, sovereignty, empowerment, beauty, and healing.

May it be an affirmation of LIFE, generating radiant health and longevity through all levels of consciousness.

May she awaken with this new beautiful breast fully embodying her divine feminine nature and power, allowing, clearly receiving, and naturally expressing her spiritual gifts and wisdom with grace and ease.

May she experience loving resonance and harmony with her mother, a relationship based on choice, liberation, and the present.

She is claiming her divine heritage as the Lady of the Lake.

So be it.

Blessed be.

During the surgery, for a few minutes, my heart began beating irregularly. This created a fear in the OR—additional heart monitors were placed on me, my family was alerted, and I wore an electrocardiogram monitor for twenty-four hours in the hospital. When my mom heard this, her first thought was that I was having a deep spiritual experience and that I was fine. This was profound for me to hear later because it confirmed that she was clearly connected to my experience during the surgery.

These are the words I spoke when I came out:

I felt abundant energy in the room.

I felt Archangel Saamprael holding me as I went into an immeasurably deep space, out of my body. I "left" and entered another realm, where I could observe what was happening around me.

Spirit doctors in Avalon had set up a grid around the hospital room, and I could feel brilliant light illuminating the space and light structures in the room.

I felt a temple above me with white pillars of light. All around were familiar beings from Avalon.

My essence shot up through the temple like a pyramid of light—I entered Avalon, where there was an initiation ceremony for me during which I became one with the Lady of the Lake.

We bathed in the lake, and she anointed me, lightly rubbing frankincense oil on my feet and forehead.

She dressed me in a purple and sapphire blue robe that matched the one she wore. She gently placed a bejeweled and radiant crown—that looked just like hers—upon my head. My feet were bare.

She escorted me into the circle of energy that she held. I merged with her. It was as though I walked into her, into the vision of her that I've been holding, and I became one with her. And realized that I am that vision—I am She.

I observed many people I knew. Kathy Jones was there, my teacher, standing at the edge of the ceremony, with a beautiful rattle and cloak. Her head was uncovered so I could fully see her face as she stood there with her arms out, between the ceremony and the barge.

Kathy beckoned me toward the boat, saying, "Now it's your turn. Are you up for it? Do you say yes?" And I said, "Yes," and stepped back onto the barge.

I continued telling the story of my experience while under anesthesia:

I felt as though a funnel was streaming down from my breast. Black smoke, and residue, like tree sap, was emerging from it, releasing from it.

There were written words and stories pouring out of indeterminate energetic shapes.

A beautiful being appeared with a magical bucket that reminded me of Blue's old purple bucket that he ate his grain from and loved so much. The bucket was catching something else also made of this indeterminate, energetic shape, almost like a cloud.

The being vanished as quickly as he'd appeared, rising up, and clearing my old wounds. All of the clearing was on the left side of my body.

I felt a karmic "board" of angels and beautiful beings, who were giving their stamp of approval for my clearing, as though they were sitting in an office. It was as though my paperwork was finished for those lessons.

I was letting go, letting go, letting it all go.

And then Archangel Saamprael, Brigid, and the Lady of the Lake appeared with their arms extended. Blue appeared, in human form, and took his place with them, also reaching his arms out to me.

Their arms reached underneath the back of my heart center, through my heart chakra as they pushed it with the energy of their hands.

A being with the ability to make herself small appeared—a Sidhe, or a Faery—another strong being. A clear stream of thick energy came out of her.

I understood they were all working together.

I heard the voice of a nurse in the background: "Are you warming up, Taylor?"

I felt the purity of Tiffany Grunwald's heart; how loving she is, and how much she respected my wishes and placed a lot of love into me.

And I felt the specialness of Chung Fu, in the pinnacle of the temple, watching over everything and saying, "Dear one, you're so courageous, and I'm so proud of you. I am here. Thank you for calling on me."

And my guide, Angelica, was there the whole time, holding my hand and literally reaching her hands into me, soothing my inner child and my "basic" self. She created a playground for my inner child, that was like the playground at Smoke Tree Ranch (where I played as a kid) with a merry-go-round.

The Lady of the Lake was still there for me, for my embodiment and return. She was playful and attentive to my inner child as well as my stronger inner maiden, who was present with her sword and shield.

I feel so strong.

I knew the karma with my mom had cleared. I knew that for that to happen, I had to have dropped into a profoundly deep space.

I'd always imagined that when visiting the karmic board, or angelic realms with the presence of my guides, I would shoot up through my crown, and move up into these higher dimensions and realms.

But I went down.

Through my root chakra, my feet, and my spine and even my low back. I dropped deeper and deeper down into a powerful place, almost into the earth.

I had to allow something to die—the old karmic burdens that I've carried from my ancestral lineage, in my maternal line, and paternal line, of women.

I saw them all in rows and performed a ceremony to release them with love. There were angels all around me as we smudged my ancestors.

Angelica said, "This is the death before the rebirth."

I saw a big book laying open, with a pen drawing a line from right to left through the page on the right side. We took it out and threw it in the fire; that transmuted it into the clearing of the karma, genetics, and everything on the ancestral line of my mother's side. Some of these, like pockets of cells and memories of patterns, were just pulled out of me, like with a little suction cup. As all was cleared, those beautiful souls were given freedom to choose where they wanted to go.

Some of them went to Avalon.

Some of the unhealthy imprints that were released weren't even from my mom; they were things she inherited that were not her true self. I could see her bathing in the lake, to release these cellular memories. When she emerged from the water, it was as though she, too, had been wiped clean.

And I forgave her. I forgave my mom, and my teenage self also forgave her.

My teenage self wants to rewrite the timeline of trauma and low self-esteem and align herself with a higher timeline, shedding the unhealthiness of the past.

And that's what she's done. I saw her before me—so pretty with her reddish brown hair.

I don't know why she didn't recognize her beauty and felt she had to dye her hair and change herself. Now she's fully alive, activated, trusting herself and her wisdom.

She's teaching me to do this, too, and making it so easy for me.

I had sunk down, almost into the earth, yet this wasn't the underworld. This was the deep layers of my consciousness.

My doctor entered the room and inquired, "Everything okay?" Ryan replied, "Yes, thank you."

Angelica was there again, and Mary Magdalene and Yeshua. The book appeared again, flipped to a very specific page. Mary Magdalene read aloud from it, and then an old samurai man appeared. He had a long gray beard and a huge table filled with knives and swords.

There were energy currents around that connected to the past. Not the past in a linear fashion, but instead timelines that are side by side and lifetimes that are side by side. Everything was present simultaneously. There was no backwards and forwards; all was present in this different dimensional space.

As Mary Magdalene read, the old man lifted up his sword and brought it down fast and then a "swoosh" sound as he cut through these energy currents connected to the past. The energy rose into the air like a gossamer thread emerging from the book, then it turned purple-y and disintegrated. A rainbow-colored energy took its place. Mary Magdalene read about taking on burdens that weren't mine—anger from my mom; anger that had been passed down to her through our lineage. A particular pattern of suppression, of trying to fit in a box, behavior that didn't belong to me, but belonged instead to my grandmother and great-grandmother through a long line of suppressing.

I just have to remember that I'm from Venus, from another star system. This work is about healing my feminine line. The sword was cutting away old karmas and burdens with profound love. And releasing it.

As I was being blessed, and healed, so were my mom, my grandmother, and all my ancestors and descendants.

My soul traveled to Venus for a few minutes to allow for this deep reconfiguration. I could see specific things being cleared, the burdens being lifted, rewritten, recoded, and reconfigured in my soul. It was a long way for me to travel but I had to go there, I traveled through a stargate and could only be there for a few minutes.

Now the Lady of the Lake, the Lady of Avalon, Brigid, and Archangels Saamprael and Michael were holding me in their powerful and loving energy. Sekhmet guarded the gates between my body in the hospital room and my soul in Venus.

The room was illuminated with loving beings, including the Spirit doctors of Avalon who were there working through my doctors.

HEALING THE MOTHER WOUND

As I lay in the hospital bed later that night, several hours after the procedure, I listened to the recording and heard my voice describe the awe-inspiring, mystical journey of healing and initiation that I had passed through during my surgery. I then handed the headphones to my mom. In a clearer state, I may have been worried about hurting her feelings. Thankfully, I was still very woozy from the medication that allowed me to share without inhibitions. Later, my mom told me that listening to my experience struck a chord of truth so deep within her that she understood herself, her life, and the choices she had made up until that time more clearly. *Praise Goddess!* I have since felt a palpable shift in our relationship and in the energy of my entire mother line. I am able to receive my mother's love and caring in a more natural and authentic way than ever before.

Dr. Grunwald came to visit me the day after surgery to tell me that the OR was completely silent as she read my prayer, and that everyone was incredibly moved. She felt inspired to offer my prayer to all her mastectomy patients, and asked if she could say a less personal version for other women. I sent her this special prayer that can be used for any woman:

Prayer for Warrior Goddesses Experiencing a Mastectomy

May this implant be tuned perfectly to the harmony of _____'s body.

May it be filled with divine love, sacredness, empowerment, beauty, and healing.

May it be an affirmation of life, generating radiant health and longevity through all levels of her consciousness.

May she awaken with this new, beautiful breast fully embodying her divine feminine nature and power, receiving and giving equally, and expressing her unique gifts and wisdom with grace and ease.

So be it. Blessed be.

A few months later, I went to see Tselem and Teraphim and spoke to them about my choice to have the mastectomy. I told them about my experience under anesthesia and about traveling to Venus. They nodded in complete acknowledgment and understanding, aware of the stargate I traveled through to get there. Tselem said keeping my nipple was very significant. Spiritually, the reason I kept it was so that I would be able to fully receive the Goddess, through the left nipple and breast, which is the feminine space of receiving. The right side is about the energy of giving. I needed this divine feminine energy from Venus, the pure feminine source of goddess energy, to completely clear and dissolve any disingenuous, misguided, distorted, or negative energy residue from past lives in which I had power over people or took power from people. Specifically, lifetimes during which I practiced dark witchcraft, manipulating energies according to personal will rather than aligning with Divine will and that which is for the highest good of all concerned.

Now, in my present life, my soul is ready to serve from a place of purity, and the purification of my vessel forced any remaining karmic material to surface, which was then completely cleared through Venus during the surgery. Tselem added that during my journey, my soul began to calibrate to the energy of Venus, which was confusing for my body. This was the reason for the irregular heartbeat.

SESSION WITH CHUNG FU, ONE MONTH AFTER MASTECTOMY SURGERY

I began by telling Chung Fu that my husband recorded about thirty-five minutes of me talking about my incredible journey while I was under anesthesia.

"You were there, Chung Fu. On the recording, I described an initiation I underwent in Avalon, and the healing of my mother line. I talked about my mother's anger, and about learning that it wasn't actually hers but from an ancestor four generations before her, and the ways it had been passed along up until now when it was being cleared. I spoke of traveling far to Venus to receive new light codes in my body. It was extraordinary that I talked about this journey with such clarity."

Chung Fu: *Yes, beloved, I was there at the ceremony on the inner plane.*

"I remember you said you were so proud of me," I said. "I felt really proud of myself for moving through the ceremony with grace, and making it beautiful, empowering myself through it. Four and a half weeks have passed since then, and I'm cancer free. This is my *official* moment of being cancer free.

"The surgery was on my mother's birthday. Afterward, she listened to the recording and heard me talking about healing my mother line, and about her anger. I think because I was still between the worlds, and highly medicated, I thought it was a good idea to ask my mom to listen to the recording. I remember saying, 'Mom, you have to hear this.' She listened to the whole thing in the hospital and felt it allowed her to see and understand her life through new eyes."

INANNA'S ASCENT

Gate 5: Retrieval of the Gold Bracelet:
Embodying My Power

As Inanna ascends through the fifth gate of the underworld, the gateway of the solar plexus that is connected to personal power, she retrieves her gold bracelet. As she places it on her wrist, she recognizes that it is no longer a symbol of her power. She has retrieved the disowned aspects of herself that had lain dormant, lost in the shadows of the underworld. She has faced her darkness, represented by her sister, Ereshkigal, embracing all that she has been, all shame, any misuse of energy, or misunderstanding. Embracing her darkness has allowed her to become fully present in her body, giving her the gift of truly knowing herself. She can feel her power pulsing in her blood and her bones, and her skin glows with starlight. The gold bracelet on her wrist was a reminder of this power, yet she knows the true source is within, and could not be truly represented in any object. Adorning herself with the gold bracelet is an act of pleasure and self-love. She knows that when she is honoring her truth within that, her will *is* the Divine will. She is in alignment with her divine nature. Inanna and I both reside in our personal authority and sovereignty as we remember the Divine Mother love that pulses in our blood.

It was through the removal of my breast that my power returned to me through the transmission of goddess love from Venus as the representation of Inanna in the heavens. I was cleansed of the suppression of my mother line so that I could receive the ancestral power that will support me moving forward. I was filled with sacred feminine love not through giving birth to a baby, but through surrendering the possibility of experiencing giving birth through this body.

When I realized I couldn't have a baby because of the risk after having an estrogen-driven cancer, I was absolved of cultural pressures to express my femininity in a certain way. Cultural pressures I didn't even realize were there until they weren't. My femininity was not contained in my breast, restricted to any particular role, and could never be objectified. My potential for feminine expression is limitless. As I ascend through the fifth gate of the underworld, I claim my gold bracelet to remind myself of the infinite source of my power, flowing through the circular, spiraling stargate portal from Venus, directly from the heart and womb of the Great Mother of All.

JOURNAL ENTRY

The first night at home after surgery, I dreamed I had a wonderful, scholarly teacher who was teaching me the initiation rites of the cult of Aphrodite/Venus, as well as ancient Pictish knowledge and language from the Picts, who were an old tribe of Scotland.

I also dreamed I was skiing and had rented equipment from a big guy like Hagrid from Harry Potter. Everyone was ahead of me on a big excursion. I didn't have any poles and was trying to catch up. There were magical people along the way giving me directions.

JOURNAL PROMPT

What does embodiment mean to you? How would it feel to be fully present in your body? What might shift in your life if you were in complete alignment with your divine nature?

MEDITATION

Sit comfortably with your spine straight, or lie down, where you will not be disturbed. Close your eyes, and begin taking in deep diaphragmatic breaths, in through the nose, filling and expanding the belly, and out through the mouth with an audible exhale...ahhh. Repeat three times.

Bringing your awareness to your solar plexus, visualize a glowing ball of light, golden and warm like the sun, shining in the center of your body. With your breath, see rays of this light expanding outward to illuminate your entire body and energy field. Every cell is being bathed in this radiant light now. Notice any shifts that occur within you as this light penetrates through the deepest levels of your body and consciousness. If there are any areas of your body that need some extra attention, place your hands there and allow this warm golden light to flood in.

This is the eternal light of your divinity, filling you with the remembrance of your divine nature. As you continue to breathe, feel the presence of this light expanding outward all around you until you are bathed in a pillar of light. This is your personal pillar of light, holding and supporting you, bringing you into alignment with your divine nature and power. The more you practice this visualization, the stronger the pillar will become, and you will experience a greater sense of presence and alignment in your life.

Take a moment now to fill your pillar of light with your prayers, intentions, and highest desires.

Inanna stands before you, offering you a gold bracelet, a symbol of the circle of light that has formed around you. As you cross the fifth gate of the underworld, you feel in resonance and alignment with the divine power that is guiding your life, holding you in grace and protection.

Breathe into your personal pillar of light a few more times, anchoring this visual in your mind. When you are ready, open your eyes and journal any insights that came forward.

Blessed be.

Chapter Eleven

REBIRTH

FOURTH GATE: VULNERABILITY

"Where there's fear, there is power."

~ Starhawk

IT'S NOT ABOUT THE FUTURE, IT'S ABOUT THE PAST

Dr. Funk had decided to remove the three lymph nodes that had tumor in them, so that all physical material in my body that had cancer would be removed. This would take the possibility of radiation off the table, or so I thought. After surgery, I learned she had removed thirteen lymph nodes, a wide circumference around the area where the tumor had been. I couldn't help but notice the sacred feminine code being revealed through the number thirteen; there are thirteen twenty-eight-day moon cycles in one year. The unnatural configuration of the Gregorian calendar has built an invisible barrier in modern society, removing us from an organic, embodied understanding of the cycles of the sun and moon. The word moon is the etymological origin of the word month, and as the Gregorian calendar is made up of twelve months, we are unknowingly divorced from the thirteenth moon.

Because the thirteenth moon is in the shadows of the unknown, it holds an association with the dark goddess. Having thirteen lymph nodes removed whispered to me of a time on the Earth when we were attuned to the harmonies of the solar and lunar cycles, and I felt a signaling from my ancestors that the wounds that had been passed down to me were now extracted from the shadows of our collective unconscious. Those lymph nodes were biopsied, and I was devastated to learn that after the chemo there was still residual tumor in those lymph nodes at the time of surgery, which meant radiation was necessary after all. I felt as though I had been rising from the dark, cold, uninhabited depths of the ocean and was beginning to see streams of light penetrating the water above me, when suddenly, I was yanked at the ankle, pulled down by the monster I had just escaped from, and forced further down into the abyss. An incredible amount of fear began to surface: fear for my life, the threat of cancer returning, and questioning how I would ever be able to live beyond the shadows of these fears. I lay in bed with drainage tubes coming out of my side, taped breasts, and a tight postsurgical bra, viscerally feeling the pain of never being able to bear a child in my body. The doctors had been telling me for months that it was way too risky for a woman with estrogen-driven cancer to have the increased estrogen in her body that would occur during pregnancy. One doctor even referred to estrogen as "cancer fuel."

I had heard all of these things on some level; however, I hadn't fully taken them in. Somewhere, I was clinging to the belief that this wasn't true for me. The shock of being completely derailed from the path I'd envisioned for my life and marriage had prevented me from really hearing my doctors. The shock had also protected me, allowing me to process the emotional material in layers.

During the time I was recovering from surgery, a dear friend gave birth to her first child. As I lay in bed wearing my postmastectomy bra, I received a text from her sharing how she was doing and expressing how painful breastfeeding was. As I read her message, I felt my heart shatter with loss, my body overcome with grief that was beyond the experiences of my personal life, or any one woman's life for that matter. This was collective grief, old grief, the pain of all the women before me who could not bear their own children. These were ancient, profound feelings of loss. I sobbed from my guts, holding my numb chest. All I could think was: *what a privilege to feel the pain of breastfeeding.*

I needed to talk to Chung Fu. As usual, he responded to the depth of grief I shared with him.

Chung Fu: *There's not really a "back to normal" after cancer. Things aren't quite the same. You always live with cancer in a certain way. It's been there, left its calling card, and it can come again.*

"I feel like I will be taking measures to prevent it for the rest of my life," I said.

It's a consciousness that's rampant in the world. There are so many types of cancer and the kind you got is from an internal source. With some cancers, you can move your physical location and the source of pollution, toxicity, or the presence of carcinogens is removed, so you remove the danger. When the source comes from within your body, your makeup and hormones, it's coming from inside you emotionally. You've worked really hard on the emotional aspect of your cancer. That's why you have to be the realist you've come to be in reducing any risks you can so you don't walk back into the danger and trigger it. You're making wise choices, but it's hard.

You are growing extraordinary courage. Feeling fear simultaneously isn't a contradiction because that's also where you are. You may have a breast implant, but you also have implants of spiritual courage and a new part of you that's coming in to deal with this, beloved. This is a part that hasn't appeared before now because the sovereign queen part of you hasn't been needed until now. This process is extensive, from lifetimes of power being taken away from you, and loss, grief. This is no small thing—it's a big turnaround, but you're doing it.

It might look as though you're afraid of cancer—and of your death in the future. But at this level, you can't feel fear about an imagined future. It's not about the future, it's about the past. It's what is in you that is moving through you. Remember what's actually happening in your body. These things are clearing; let them clear. Go to the tears, let the tears come. Let the fear shake you. But don't believe it. Don't believe with your mind that it's about the future. Your body is full of the past, dear one. It can't be full of the future; you haven't created that yet. You are free. You are creating the future of your desire. Understand it, look at it. Look at what you've done, what you're accomplishing— you're clearing the past from your body.

His words resonated so clearly as my truth. I could feel myself calming inside.

This is ancient work. In one sense, you've had no option but to trans-form or die. I include the word "die" because of the pattern of terror you have been dealing with. Terror that was suppressed by the drugs you were forced to take as a young girl. The terror of being stopped from becoming your true self. You held this terror tightly in your body. Now you're moving through the deep levels from before the time you were stopped from becoming yourself. You're moving through a psychic, spir-itual death and through the ultimate stopping of a woman's power by killing her. You're resurrecting your power. You're bringing back parts of you that have never had a chance to exist in this life. As you con-quer these hurdles, you bring your higher Self, your priestess self, your goddess self, back. Each time, you reclaim a new level of your power. A deeper level of your freedom. A deeper level of your divine presence.

Keep going on this journey, and don't stop the flow of tears. Don't get caught up in placing your fear into the future. It's not about the future. It's old. Say, "Thank Goddess, thank you; take this fear, it's old. I'm done with it. Thank you for showing it to me. It's wracking my body. Just like the way I was tortured and killed slowly, and everything taken from me. I give it to you. I give all these old memories to you. I give all of these old experiences to you."

Understand that these conditions are bringing out your deepest fears. This may feel as though the conditions are causing you fear you never felt you had, but the fears have been sitting there for a very long time—for lifetimes, actually. This is the first lifetime in which you've returned with enough courage, experience, wisdom, and personal power to do this work.

No ordinary person could have done the work you've done, or carried it all the way through. It takes someone of power to do this. You know it; you can feel it. And every time you're challenged, just keep remembering, "That is me coming back. I'm back. I'm returning to do this. This is my life; this is my body. I'm changing my body because I can."

Chung Fu's wise insight brought me balance, comfort, and courage. His perspective helped me to release the debilitating grip of fear I had been living with since the news that I'd have to endure radiation after all. I hung up the phone after our session feeling gratitude for the wise teachers that Goddess had brought into my life.

GOING BACKWARD

There was a summertime heat wave in Glastonbury, and my friend Carrie and I walked in the blazing sun to Bride's Mound, a lesser-known sacred site connected with the goddess Brigid. I have always felt comforted by the land in this enchanted place; it resonates with pure healing energy. Carrie and I lay on the earth in silence for a bit and then I asked if she would like to call in the wheel, which is particularly potent to do out on the land. We rose to our feet. As part of my daily practice, I call in the wheel every morning and night, inviting the energies of the goddesses into my day and giving thanks for the blessings they bring to my life. The flow of the directions is ingrained in my being.

It was the end of July, the time of Lammas, the mother goddess, whose direction is the southwest. I began by calling to the Great Mother, invoking Her qualities of nurturing, tender loving care, and Her abundant nature. Instead of turning to the right, to the west, as I have done for years, I instinctively turned left and began calling in the mother of water, Domnu, and the Lady of the Lake, from the south. Not until I started turning left again, to the southeast, did it dawn on me—*I'm going backward!* I said this to Carrie in disbelief, and the moment the words came out of my mouth I felt *I must be unwinding something.* I shared this with Carrie and said, "I'm going to trust this," and continued to move around counterclockwise.

In energy healing practices, moving counterclockwise unwinds and clears energy, while clockwise sends and empowers energy. I continued to move counterclockwise, to Rhiannon in the southeast, Artha in the east, Brigid in the northeast, and Danu in the north. When I turned to the northwest, the direction of the dark goddess, the crone, Keridwen, and Sheela-Na-Gig, something phenomenal happened. I felt anxiety building in my chest and instantly was overcome with the fear of something else bad happening. The fear and stress that I had become accustomed to living with was devouring me, again. The feeling was building and as I began to cave into myself, I released a huge burp from my chest. I fell to my knees and cried, my body heaving into the earth. I was engulfed in darkness and immediately felt myself in the underworld cave I had been in for so many months, and Keridwen was there. She looked at me, the fierce grandmother, and with great intensity and sternness in her eyes said, "You can go now; I'm done with you." I felt a profound release, as if a rubber band that had been tightly wrapped to my chest was cut free. We stared at each other for a moment, her eyes gleaming in solidarity, in recognition of my warrior journey. She gave me a loving grandmotherly hug, and without a moment's hesitation, I turned to leave.

I walked briskly through the dark, following a tunnel, and began to see faint light up ahead. I found myself in a familiar place, and as I got closer to the light, I realized I was exiting through West Kennett Long Barrow, and that part of me had been there since my Samhain ceremony just days before Blue's passing and weeks before being diagnosed. During that ceremony, I had led a vision journey to meet the dark goddess, traveling through the passage of West Kennett Long Barrow to meet Keridwen in her medicine cave. *I have been there all this time.* West Kennett Long Barrow is a powerful, ancient Neolithic site. A barrow is another word for tomb, and is known to be a place of tomb and womb, death and rebirth. Ancient people used it ceremonially, and as a place of burial. There is a circular womb-like cave in the innermost chamber, and a dark passageway with pathways to small chambers off to each side. At the entrance there is a line of standing stones. West Kennett Long Barrow is aligned to true east. In my priestess tradition, the east is the place of rebirth. On this day, I walked through the passageway and out around the standing stones, finding myself standing on the earth at dusk.

A waxing crescent moon is rising and the earth is cool beneath my feet. I gently shiver and become aware of my clothing, tattered and covered in dirt and mud, as is the rest of my body. I notice Keridwen's hawk flying above me, and I begin walking down the hillside toward the nearby Avebury stone circles. With the hawk as my guide, I arrive at the processional line of standing stones, and feel led to touch a particular stone. Suddenly, I feel as if I'm on a moving train, and I know the hawk will alert me to which stop is mine. He telepathically directs me to another stone, and in a vortex of moving energy, I feel myself being carried away. The atmosphere changes and

I see myself bathing in the waters of the White Spring in Glaston-bury, holy waters that emerge from the earth beneath the Tor, an area known to be an entry point to the underworld, or for me today, an exit point. I bathed in these cool waters and cleansed the dirt and mud of the underworld from my body. The water was startlingly cold, and as I instinctively drew in a deep breath, I became aware of my forehead pressed upon the earth, my body curled over my knees, and I felt Carrie's loving hand on my back. I had been given the gift of rebirth.

As I breathed a sigh of relief, I realized once again the level of fear and stress I had become accustomed to. Just as soldiers normalize bullets flying by their heads as they fight in battle, I was in a constant state of bracing myself for impact in the form of heart-wrenching news or frightening statistics about my survival. It had been com-pletely debilitating. I began to see the process of unwinding ahead of me, understanding this journey has a divine timing of its own that cannot be rushed. There was unwinding from the trauma and crisis, from any lingering ideas of going "back" to my life before cancer. There was releasing the toxins from my body, the grief from my heart, and the imprints of fear from the medical community. I wanted to spin and spin, and like a child playfully turning circles in this meadow, spin counterclockwise and unwind it all. I knew it would be an ongoing process to stabilize and integrate my transformation.

Before my experience with cancer, when I heard people speak of spiritual initiation and being tested by Goddess, I felt frightened. I think subconsciously I knew that the testing I would endure would be significant. After being released from the underworld, I felt pro-found joy and gratitude for having completed the journey, and also for having the courage to embark on it in the first place. Living a life in service to Goddess requires deep surrender and a willing-ness to be taken on an initiatory journey. Resistance to this process creates blockages, obstacles, and overall, more suffering and confu-sion. I realized no matter how hard I tried to will myself out of the underworld, it was not going to happen until Goddess released me from her grip. She brought me into that cave to show me the depths of my shadow, my fears, and to face my mortality, and release all misidentifications about who I am. It was a process of purification on all levels. Now it was time to rise into the light of day and slowly emerge into the world, bringing with me all the wisdom from my time in the dark. The next day, I went to the White Spring and cleansed in the water, stating my intention aloud to wash the underworld from me. Weaving images from our inner world into the outer world and vice versa builds bridges in consciousness to travel beyond the boundaries of the mind.

INANNA'S ASCENT

Gate 4: She Retrieves Her Breastplate: Vulnerability

As Inanna makes her way out of the underworld, she retrieves her breastplate at the fourth gate of the heart. This gateway is the bridge between the upper and lower energy centers of the body, connecting the lower three chakras to the upper three. Her body is now clothed in her royal robe, and she carries her lapis measuring rod and wears her gold bracelet, the adornments corresponding with her lower energy centers. As she enters the territory of her heart, she contemplates the healing that has occurred. When she entered the underworld, her heart had been cracked open, revealing grief and pain that the breastplate covering had hidden and protected. The breastplate had enabled her to remain closed to the full expression of her life, as at that time, she had related only to the conditions of the upper world. Its removal allowed the medicine of the underworld to penetrate her and flow through the cracks, releasing grief and fear, bringing her closer to joy and freedom. The breastplate no longer protects her from being vulnerable, but instead reminds her of the healing that occurs through embracing vulnerability.

As I walk through the fourth gate of the underworld, I reflect on how raw and exposed I felt when confronted with my fear of not being liked or approved of by others, and my need to be seen a certain way to value myself. My journey through the underworld has taught me ferocity. Like a lioness who fiercely protects and tends her young, I protect and tend to the needs of the younger parts of myself that I have reclaimed. I listen deeply to the needs of my heart, honoring the resounding truth that my heart emits. Being ferocious has nothing to do with anyone else; it's about having the courage to truly honor oneself, despite what others may think. It's about understanding that the best I can do is act in accordance with my heart; everything else is beyond my control.

The word courage comes from the Latin root "cor," which means "heart." One of the earliest definitions of courage was "to speak one's mind by telling all one's heart." I learned this when I was twenty-five and was so moved by it that I had the word "heart" tattooed on my left wrist. As I retrieve my breastplate and place it over my chest, I place my left hand to my heart, receiving the full wisdom that my spirit had been hinting at to my younger self when she had the impulse to get that tattoo. My heart is etched with courage. My self-worth comes from living from my heart.

JOURNAL ENTRY

I woke up in the middle of the night and couldn't go back to sleep. I was feeling dread at going in for chemo the next day. Even though this will be my last round, I absolutely don't want to do this. I want to recover and begin the process of emerging from the underworld. I can feel how much closer I am. Thinking back to the beginning of this journey and the intense darkness, sadness, and fear I was walking through, facing the unknown—those days when I could not stop sobbing in despair and fear all day long. There's a type of crying that feels cathartic, and a type of primal guttural crying that is very painful, and the place of despair and grief I was tapping into was beyond the depths of any feeling I had previously even come close to, or even knew was possible.

What a classic initiatory journey this has been. Descending at Samhain and emerging at Beltane. When I woke last night in my half-sleep state, I was receiving healing from my guides, helpers, and Spirit doctors—thank you! I felt a big clearing and cord cutting. I also repeated my Louise Hay mantras and felt Archangel Muriel with diamond light all through my body, and was then surrounded by a rainbow aura.

I am grateful for the time I've been able to be fully focused on healing. I haven't driven a car or been anywhere in public (aside from being driven to doctors) for almost five months. I wonder how it will feel to emerge and be reborn.

JOURNAL PROMPT

Contemplate the phrase "perfect vulnerability." What would it mean to live life in perfect vulnerability? What is the truth of your heart?

MEDITATION

Sit comfortably with your spine straight, or lie down, where you will not be disturbed. Close your eyes, and begin taking in deep diaphragmatic breaths, in through the nose, filling and expanding the belly, and out through the mouth with an audible exhale...ahhh. Repeat three times.

Bring your hands to your heart space. As you breathe in and out, practice simultaneously giving and receiving love to yourself. Feel the flow of loving energy moving from your hands into your heart and from your heart back into your hands. Become attuned to the presence of unconditional love that resides here.

Visualize a treasure chest resting within this sacred space of your heart. Receive the beauty of this chest. What material is it made from? What embellishments or carvings does it have? Take a moment to observe the treasure chest of your heart.

See Inanna standing before you, holding a key. This key was retrieved in the underworld, after the breastplate had been dissolved. Inanna places the key in your hand, and you unlock and open the chest. Light streams out from the center as the treasure of your heart is revealed.

What do you see or feel? Allow yourself to receive the beauty that is revealed to you. Perhaps you see colorful jewels or symbols, or perhaps you experience a quality or feeling. Trust whatever comes forward.

Experience the energy of the open treasure chest filling your heart with greater levels of loving presence. The gift of your open heart allows you to authentically share your inner beauty with the people in your life. The treasure that has been revealed allows you to trust that you are safe to share from a place of vulnerability, knowing that your deepest heart's desires are messages from your soul, showing you what is possible.

Take in a few deep breaths, feeling love and gratitude for your open heart.

When you are ready, open your eyes and journal any insights that came forward.

Blessed be.

Chapter Twelve

RISE

THIRD GATE: FINDING
MY TREASURE

"Let my worship be within the heart that rejoices, for behold,
all acts of love and pleasure are my rituals."

~ Doreen Valiente, "Charge of the Star Goddess"

OUTER HEALING: WALKING THE LABYRINTH

During the season of Ostara, the time of the spring equinox, I began to have a visceral feeling of new power rising in me. I was simultaneously training as a Priestess of the Goddess while undergoing the many pieces of medical treatment, completing assignments in the moments I could summon enough energy. The healing journey seemed to be part of my training, as though everything was woven together. One of our assignments during this second spiral was to create three public goddess-centered events or ceremonies. For self-preservation, I had been living in a state of isolation, so my teacher, Luna, suggested that one of my events be invitation-only with my prayer circle sisters. This was perfect for me.

· · ·

There are eight of us gathered at my friend Val's home. We sit together in the shape of a half moon, with Baelyn, who is serving us ceremonial tea, in the center. The practice of Cha Dao, or the way of tea, has been a personal practice for several years. In 2011, my then-boyfriend Colin and I embarked on a divinely guided adventure through Asia, where we discovered an ancient tea tradition and befriended a tea master in Taiwan. We were so deeply moved and inspired by our experiences with tea that upon returning home we opened a teahouse in Venice, California, called Temple Tea. The practice of Cha Dao flowed into the hearts and homes of many, beginning with our friends and expanding into a community that continues to blossom today. Sitting for tea ceremony creates a beautiful opportunity for experiencing inner stillness; washing away the busyness of the outside world, dropping into the heart, and receiving Mother Earth's love. Together at Val's home, we sit in silence, sipping bowls of earthy pu-erh tea, grounding into sacred space together. After some heartfelt and tearful sharing, we collect our things and head off to a nearby hiking trail. Shaking rattles, gently beating drums, and humming softly, we make our way up the trail. After about a mile of walking, which is quite an achievement for me in the midst of cancer treatment, we come to a labyrinth built of stone on a bluff overlooking the Pacific Ocean. It is wonderful to be out in nature, breathing fresh air. I remove the wool cap from my head and close my eyes as the ocean breeze cleanses my hairless crown. Gathering leaves, stones, and materials from the land, along with crystals I have brought with me, I begin building an altar on the earth near the labyrinth. One sister is cleansing everyone with incense while another sister is holding a rhythmic drumbeat. Removing my shoes to feel my bare feet on the cool earth, I guide everyone in a clockwise direction around the outside edge of the labyrinth, forming a circle. Clockwise, or sunwise, is the traditional way to enter a ceremonial space, a stone circle, or a sacred well. When I was in Ireland, I learned to approach a holy well by walking around it three times clockwise.

Standing in a circle around the labyrinth, looking at the faces of the women who have loved and held me in this journey, with the glimmering blue ocean as our backdrop, I feel overcome with gratitude. I guide everyone through a grounding meditation, visualizing a beam of light descending down from their root center, between their legs, connecting down to the iron core crystal in the heart of Mother Earth. Feeling the unconditional love and support of Mother Earth, we breathe this energy in, inviting it into our hearts.

From the heart center, I invite everyone to bring their awareness up to their crowns, where a second beam of light is ascending up through the sky and into the heavens, connecting with their mother star, a star that burns just for them. This starlight flows down through the sparkling beam of light into their hearts, filling them with celestial energy and the love of their higher selves, angels, guides, and spiritual support systems. Together, we breathe the earth and the stars into our hearts.

I begin to call in the Wheel of Bridannia. The wind picks up and I consciously project my voice as loud as I can, yet I'm surprised at its volume. This voice doesn't feel as though it's coming from my fatigued body, but from somewhere else. As I've gotten closer to the end of treatment, the cumulative effect of chemo has really set in, and I've recently experienced days in which I've lost my voice. Today, though, I feel my ancient priestess self within, her voice booming through me. Her presence is rising from the depths of my being, like a snake rising up from a hole in the earth.

After calling in the wheel, we are ready to walk into the labyrinth. The labyrinth is a powerful healing tool that can help with releasing patterns from consciousness and creating new ones. As we enter, the invitation is to focus on letting go of a particular pattern or behavior. When walking out of the labyrinth, the invitation is to envision what we would like to put in place of our old behavior to weave a new pathway into our consciousness. As we walk in, I ask my sisters to hold a collective intention of releasing all dis-ease from my body, as well as any place in my consciousness that the dis-ease is connected. I ask that as we walk out, they visualize me in radiant health and wholeness, aligned with my high Self, my ancient priestess self, and my young maiden priestess self, who is expressing all her magical gifts, including "Sight." Silently, we walk in one by one, everyone breathing deeply, drumming, and rattling.

I am standing in the center as all of my sisters quietly surround me. With a spontaneous burst of energy, we all begin to shout and moan, releasing sound as the drumbeats get louder and louder. A palpable energy swirls around us as we release primal noises from our open mouths. We are in a collective energy field, being moved together. The screams, moans, and shouts shift into laughter, our bodies trembling in the presence of such powerful energy.

Returning to a moment of silence, one of my friends begins singing, "My body is a living temple of love, my body is a living temple of love, my body is the body of the Goddess, my body is the body of the Goddess," and as we join in the song, each woman moves forward and places her hands on my left breast. I feel their love, prayers, and support pouring into my body. A vortex of energy spirals around us and I am at the center, all the healing love being transmitted directly into my left breast. The repetition of the song lulls us into a peaceful trance, always one of my favorite moments in ritual. I love the use of song to shift states of consciousness. Our collective energy field is building and our consciousness is shifting so that we may get out of our own way, allowing Spirit to move through us, to enter our sacred space and respond to our prayers. The lyrics of the song change to:

> *My breast is a living temple of love. My breast is a*
> *living temple of love...*
>
> *My breast is the breast of the Goddess.*

Singing together makes us all tear up and soon those tears are flowing, our eyes sparkling in recognition of the magic beyond this world that is communing with us. We join hands in a circle and begin to sing my healing song:

I am in absolute devotion

To my divinity

I am

The living spirit within

I am

The living embodiment of the Goddess

I am

The Lady of the Lake

Lady of the Lake, rise

Lady of the Lake, rise

Lady of the Lake, rise!

As I sing, "I am the Lady of the Lake," my friends sing, "My sister Taylor, the Lady of the Lake!" And together we belt out, "Lady of the Lake, rise! Lady of the Lake, rise! Lady of the Lake, *rise!*"

Blissfully, we walk out of the labyrinth, buzzing with energy. I had intended for everyone to make a second personal walk through the labyrinth to speak prayers for themselves, and I mention this to my sisters. My sister Baelyn replies, "Your healing is our healing," and everyone wholeheartedly agrees. This feels magnificent. The sun is setting over the brilliant ocean as we emerge from our ceremony and walk back down the trail at dusk.

. . .

After this gorgeous ritual and labyrinth walk, we returned to Val's home where we sat around the fire and ate dinner. When we finished eating, I brought out a sacred medicine bundle I had created with some of my hair. I knew I wanted to save the majority of my hair to throw into a bonfire in Glastonbury and was working up to that. We passed the bundle around along with some sage, rosemary, and rose petals, and everyone added herbs to the bag, along with their blessings for my healing and transformation. As a friend drummed, I offered this medicine bundle into the fire. The perfect way to end a beautiful, magical day.

. . .

Six weeks after surgery, the earliest time I could possibly fly, I got on a plane to England. Every summer there is a Goddess Conference in Glastonbury, and I knew that I wanted to burn my hair in the annual bonfire.

I'm standing with a group of my priestess sisters, priest brother, and two dear prayer circle sisters, Ashley and Val, who traveled to meet me in Glastonbury. I'm wearing a silver cloak in honor of my maiden self, who appeared wearing silver in my visions. My hair has grown in about half an inch. I stand before the fire holding a ball of dry, tangled hair in my hands, the hair that was shaved from my head nine months ago. I begin naming aloud all the things I am releasing into this fire to be transmuted—all pain, negativity, dis-ease, fragmentation, fear, suppression, withholding—I see them gone. I hold the hair in front of my heart, visualizing all remnants of these energies being released into the hair that represents my old self. I extend my arms above my head, the fire blazing before me, and I shout prayers of affirmation, declaring what is true for me.

"My body is vibrantly healthy and well, filled with vitality! I am living a long, beautiful life! I am living to be a wise and wonderful crone!"

I feel the power of the words I have spoken resonating around me and "crack!"—a firework explodes in the distance. I hear my friends gasp and look at each other in bewilderment as we all shout, "Blessed be!" in celebration of the divinely timed exclamation point.

The fire is blazing and I walk as close as I can. Standing with the ball of hair in front of my chest again, I throw it, with all my might, thrusting it forward with both arms and expelling all of its energy out of me.

The smell of burnt hair swirls around us as my priestess family holds me in a group hug, whispering words of blessings: "You are living a long, beautiful, healthy life, in service to Goddess. I see you as a wise elder. You have so much to offer this world, so many gifts, so much magic to share. Your prayers have been heard and answered. You are free from dis-ease now and forever. You are so loved." I weep as I allow their loving words to enter my heart, feeling such deep relief.

About six weeks later, just before the following autumn equinox, I return to Glastonbury for my initiation as a Priestess of Goddess. There is a sacred site in Glastonbury called the Tor, a high, distinctively shaped hill that rises dramatically from the landscape and can be seen for miles in all directions. There is a large tower dedicated to St. Michael on top of the hill, which was built in the fourteenth century.

St. Michael was known as the dragon slayer, and the Tor is known as having a convergence of powerful ley lines, earth currents also known as dragon lines, flowing beneath it. The first time my bare feet merged with this powerful earth, I felt an electrifying surge beneath me that was unmistakable. In an attempt to usurp this sacred pagan site, Christians built St. Michael's tower at the apex of the hill. Taking over ancient power spots dedicated to Goddess was common practice for Christians all over Europe. The old ways were so deeply ingrained in the collective belief systems that the Christian church tried to dominate these places and use their power for their benefit, as they were impossible to erase. Dion Fortune, a well-known occultist who lived in Glastonbury in the early 1900s, said the irony is that the tower brilliantly channels and empowers the vortex of energies converging on the Tor. I feel that, too.

The Tor is surrounded by a winding spiral path that looks like indentations in the slopes. When viewed from above, the path forms a labyrinth, an ancient symbol that can be seen in carvings from five thousand or more years ago. A labyrinth is different from a maze, with only one way in and one way out; you walk around seven layers until arriving in the center and then walk back out. The seven levels are also connected with the seven chakras. Ancient people used labyrinths as a symbolic pilgrimage. When it was much more difficult to travel, one would imagine the center as the holy place they desired to visit, and journey to the center to make offerings and speak prayers. The labyrinth path within the slopes of Glastonbury Tor is thought to be an ancient pilgrim's path. On my initiation weekend as a Priestess of Goddess, we walked this path. It takes about six hours to walk in and the same time to walk out. We walked in on Saturday and walked out on Sunday. When we arrived in the center of the labyrinth on Saturday evening, we went into our ceremony while physically and psychically in the center of the labyrinth.

INNER HEALING: BRAIDING ALL THE PARTS OF ME BACK TOGETHER

I sit in the grass, pulling my sapphire-blue cloak close as the wind blows harder. The sun is setting on our beautiful autumn day and I feel chilled. My body is exhausted and I'm wondering where the energy will come from to get through this ceremony. My face is painted with ochre. I am wearing a white dress underneath my wool cloak. After listening to some of my fellow initiates speak their dedication to the Goddess, I feel pulled to enter the center of the circle to make my vows. As I sit before the altar facing the Tor, tears begin to dampen my cheeks. *I've made it to this moment.* A vision flashes before me: I see myself during chemo, my face swollen with bright red, bleary eyes and that dreadful headscarf covering my bald head. *I've made it through.* I begin to sob, my body heaving as I let go and allow myself to fall forward toward the earth.

I don't know how much time passes before I sit up, but for a while, no words surface. I wait for them to come and hear myself thanking the Goddess for showing me who I am, for showing me the depth of my courage and strength, for helping me heal and transform, and for helping me remember Avalon. I pray for a long, radiantly healthy life so that I may be a clear channel in service to Her love and grace. My words echo in the night as I begin to speak my vows, words that will remain between my heart and Hers.

After the ceremony, I'm exhausted and almost delirious from the physical and emotional exertion. A friend drives me home and I collapse into bed. The next morning, we all meet in the center of the labyrinth on the slopes of the Tor to begin our journey out. We walk for a few hours in silence before coming upon our ceremonial site from the night before. Reverently, we gather around our altar of flowers and apples, and my eye catches something new in the center. *Is that a braid of hair?* Bewildered, I blink as I stare at an auburn-colored braid, perfectly intact, that looks as if it was cut cleanly off someone's head with a sword, lying in the center of last night's altar.

"Is that yours?" one of my sisters asks.

"I burned mine a few months ago at the Goddess Conference," I reply, in disbelief.

We all feel something special about this mysterious hair that has appeared out of nowhere. We're silent for a moment. Then, one of my sisters exclaims, "It's for you! A gift from the Lady of Avalon, a symbol of your new life! She heard you!" A wave of energy surges through me and I feel overcome with emotion—relief, joy, gratitude. I feel seen and heard, acknowledged by Goddess. I raise my arms to the sky and shout, "Yes! Thank you!" I stand in awe, reveling in the mystery of this braid, a gift from beyond the veil. In the past, my long hair had always been in a braid down my left side. More recently, the Lady of the Lake had come to me during a session with Chung Fu and shared a visual involving a braid to support my integration after all the deep soul retrieval work. In the week leading up to this ceremony, I had been walking the land visualizing a braid, imagining that I was weaving all the parts of myself back together.

MESSAGE FROM THE LADY OF THE LAKE

After the soul retrieval of my priestess self in Avalon, the Lady of the Lake spoke these words through me:

Oh, beloveds. You have both returned to me. What a blessed day. What a day of celebration that the reuniting of my two priestesses, together with me, as one, in this body, has come to pass. May we walk once more along the sacred lands, along the shores of this holy isle. And may we remember the waters, knowing they are deep within the Earth. The very same waters that we worked with so long ago. And at the same time, not so long ago. May we walk together, resting in moments of stillness and silence and, also, in celebration and ceremony. May you know, beloved, as you walk this land over these next few weeks, you are walking as three. Feel the integration of these three energies weaving into you like a braid. And feel that movement, that visual inside you, as though you are braiding hair, braiding, weaving these pieces together, and with that, you're also weaving in the threads of your brothers and sisters. Focus on that weaving, braiding yourself back together.

OUTER HEALING MIRRORS INNER HEALING

Any doubts about the miraculous nature of this were put to rest when I learned a few hours later that my teacher, Kathy, had been out walking her dog in the early morning Sunday, after the night of our ceremony, and noticed the braid as she passed by the site. She told me that upon seeing it, she knew it had something to do with me. We had left the site the night before after 10:00 p.m., and it was cold, windy, pitch dark, and there was no braid there. Then the next morning at dawn, the braid had apparently magically appeared, perfectly placed in the center. It was highly unlikely that someone was wandering around in the dark near our ceremony site, able to see our altar in the night, let alone carrying a freshly cut braid of hair! Even if that had indeed happened, I still felt the hand of Goddess guiding and directing it all.

I couldn't wait to share this with Alisha, who immediately felt the braid was a gift from the Lady of the Lake, placed from "beyond the veil." I knew intuitively that it was magically protected, and if I had touched it, it would have disintegrated. As Alisha shared her thoughts with me, I felt a kaleidoscope of my inner and outer worlds melting together in psychedelic colors and patterns. *I had dreamt of my hair disintegrating, and of my braid being cut off by a sword. The Lady of the Lake had given me a message about braiding myself back together as I walked the land.* These were visions and experiences that I had expressed solely within my journal, and here they were, appearing in my waking life. The threads within me have been woven back together, and the beauty of the tapestry is being revealed. I am rising from the ashes of the disintegrated hair—the hair that was incinerated in flames just days after I was released from the underworld; that vanished in the woods when I drank the potion from the old woman; the blonde braid that was cut off by a sword and stained with a drop of blood, now returning to me in an auburn shade, transformed by the bloodshed. This braid was a confirmation, a nod from the Divine, a symbol from the magical world passing through to the physical acknowledging, "*You did it.*" I'd found the treasure. I'd reclaimed my shadow sister from the underworld. I'd integrated the lessons, and I *am* rising.

INANNA'S ASCENT

Gate 3: Retrieves Her Strand of Beads: Finding My Treasure

As Inanna ascends through the third gate of the underworld, she retrieves the strand of beads that once hung from her neck. These beads align with her throat chakra, the energy center connected with communication. She had no voice in the underworld and was not able to communicate in the ways she was accustomed to in the upper world. When she surrendered to the ways of the underworld and opened to receive divine assistance, new energy rose to express her true voice.

As she fastens the beads around her neck, she vows to always communicate from her heart, knowing this is more powerful than speaking from her status as queen, where she might be limited by royal propriety. She will rise to her throne while leading from her divine attunement, expressing all of who she is.

As I walk through the third gate of the underworld, I reclaim the full power of my voice, remembering that my voice is the voice of the Divine. I allow all the previously unspoken words to bellow out of me, not in perfectly formed sentences, but in raw, primal, guttural screams. I've learned the language of the underworld that demanded that I let go of worry about how I sound, how others may respond, or of the need "to get it right." Remembering that I am a living embodiment of Goddess brings me a sense of safety and inherent protection. I can now freely communicate the truth of my heart, from the living spirit within.

JOURNAL ENTRY, AROUND THE TIME OF MY UNVEILING CEREMONY, SHAVING MY HEAD

Dreamed about having dark energy on my hair and needing to get rid of it. I was with a woman who was explaining this to me; she cut my

braid off with a sword. My hair had a speck of blood on it. Later, this
woman prepared a bath of black water for me to cleanse in.

JOURNAL ENTRY, MESSAGE FROM THE LADY OF THE LAKE

Beloved one, I am here to cleanse the waters of your heart, the tides of
your emotion that exist there. Allow yourself to feel my hands at your
heart emanating a healing blue light. All dis-eased, heavy, imbal-
anced, or negative emotions are being washed away and transmuted
into love. See your heart as a crystal-clear lake with beautiful, radiant
reflections of light dancing across the surface. You are clear, healthy,
whole. You are healed. It is done.

. . .

JOURNAL PROMPT

What is the language of your soul? If your soul had its own unique
song, what would it be? How would it sound?

MEDITATION

Sit comfortably with your spine straight, or lie down, where you will
not be disturbed. Close your eyes, and begin taking in deep diaphragmatic breaths, in through the nose, filling and expanding the belly,
and out through the mouth with an audible exhale...ahhh. Repeat
three times.

Bring your awareness to your throat, and visualize a sapphire-colored energy emanating outward, blue rays of light streaming in all directions. As you focus your attention in the center of your throat, you see that the source of this light is a radiant blue jewel, glowing and vibrating with energy. As you attune to the subtle vibrations arising from this jewel, you feel an innate familiarity, a sense of recognition. The jewel is actually making a sound, a gorgeous tone that resonates in the deepest levels of your memory. This radiant jewel is singing the song of your soul, the unique frequency that you and only you emit out into the universe.

Relax your face and your jaw, and open your throat to invite this frequency to move through your voice. Give yourself permission to express vocally as this energy moves through you. Do not think about how it may sound; simply open and invite this frequency to manifest through your voice. Notice any feelings that arise and flood them with the sapphire light, continuing to invite the sound to move through you.

This jewel in your throat connects you with your authentic expression, the song of your soul. Aligning with this magical jewel will infuse your communication with the vibration of your soul's light, so that all the words you speak will be carried on the frequency of the living spirit that dwells within your heart. Take a moment to visualize the words you speak in the world from this moment forward, resonating with the song of your soul. How will it feel to express your true voice?

Bring your hands to your throat as an offering of gratitude for the energy that has been cultivated there.

When you are ready, open your eyes and journal any insights that came forward.

Blessed be.

Chapter Thirteen

STEPPING INTO MY RADIANCE

SECOND GATE: I AM LIGHT

"She changes everything She touches and
Everything She touches changes
Everything lost is found again in a new form, in a new way
Everything hurt is healed again in a new time in a new day
She changes everything She touches and
Everything She touches changes."

~ Lauren Liebling and Starhawk, from a goddess chant
sung in the Reclaiming tradition

A massive wildfire broke out in Los Angeles a few days before I was scheduled to drive down to San Diego to begin radiation treatment and we were evacuated from our home. Smoke billowed over the next canyon as we drove down our street, unsure of how long we'd be gone and praying we'd be fortunate enough to have a home to return to. We stayed for a few days with friends, rooted indoors because of the visibly poor air quality. Sitting in their guest room with my cats meowing in confusion, I stared out the window at the smoke-filled world that was covered in ash. I was aware that the elemental mother of fire was beckoning me. I was preparing to endure being burned every day for five weeks, at the same time that fire was raging in the city that had held me through my healing thus far. Amid the tragic burning of the city, I knew that fire could bring an opportunity for purification. I hoped it would be the same for me. Still under mandatory evacuation orders when it came time to begin my treatment, we arrived at our rental apartment in San Diego with our two cats and the few items we had quickly thrown in a bag before leaving our home. Up to this point, I had been surrounded by my familiar altar, healing tools and creature comforts, along with the loving support of my family and sisters during various treatments. But now, I sensed there was significance in the unfamiliar territory of facing radiation alone. No one can be in the room during a radiation treatment, not even a medical technician.

I had chosen proton therapy, a form of radiation that is more targeted than standard radiation therapy for cancer. Although technically the cancer had been removed from my body during surgery, three positive lymph nodes had also been removed (meaning they still had traces of tumor in them) and this is what had warranted the radiation. This was a precaution in case there were any lingering cells connected to a lymph node pathway still in my body. Any remaining cells had been resistant to chemo, but apparently cells that are resistant to chemo will be wiped out by radiation, and vice versa. Because the chest has so many vital organs nearby, and the tumors had been on my left side, this meant there was a threat of radiation touching my heart and lung. When I was scanned for traditional radiation, it showed that my lung would receive excess radiation and potential collateral damage.

"You may have a cough for the rest of your life," the radiation oncologist said.

No, thank you. Proton therapy is still radiation; however, it delivers the radiation in a more precise and targeted way so there is less risk to surrounding organs. The only proton facility in the state that would treat me was in San Diego, so that's where we'd gone.

. . .

Five days a week for five weeks I am taken into a cold medical facility where I change into a gown that is open in the front. I lie down on a metal slab with my arms over my head, placing them into a mold of my body that positions me exactly the same way each day. My feet are bound together by a large rubber band, and I lie there topless. The techs poke and prod me until everything is precisely in place, and then quickly leave the room when they start the machine. I lie there completely alone, gripping my crystals in my hands and holding my healing visualizations in my mind, trying to keep my body as still as possible.

SESSION WITH CHUNG FU

"They're radiating my left chest up to my neck and collarbone, all over my reconstructed breast and armpit, to the center of my chest," I say. "The aim in treating my reconstructed breast is to radiate the skin and subcutaneous tissue as well as the chest wall. They want to go really deep in case there are any remaining cells that could create a recurrence in my skin, in the chest wall, or the surrounding lymph channels. This is a preventative measure."

Chung Fu: Radiation is a massive heat source created by man. Understand that you, too, are a source of light. Imagine and affirm that you are made of light. You can raise the natural solar energy of your being. Your physical body is made of matter, and its density has fallen out of the vibration of the light, taking on darkness and becoming diseased. The vast resource of light within you can energize your cells and bring them up to a vibration of power. Your light, far greater than the power of the radiation, absorbs its power. The light emanating from you commands the solar energy to come forth from Source and fill up your body.

All light comes from the sun. So, you could say that radiation is a permutation of solar energy. Fill your heart, fill your lungs, and imagine you are radiant with healthy, powerful solar light. When the radiation hits your body, your own light power will take it only to where it's been directed, only to those places where the darkness, or any dis-ease or cancer, is visible. When you fill your body with light, this makes the path carrying the dis-ease show up more clearly.

You are holding a higher quotient, a higher vibration, of the light than the radiation. The light you are holding will dissolve the radiation and protect you from receiving it in the parts of your body that don't need it. The radiation will move to those places that are a bit lower in light and may have a tiny amount of cancer because your light will reveal them. In your luminosity, those places will show up, and the radiation will go there naturally.

Breathe in the feeling that you are solar light. Breathe right into your breast, and see the sunlight coming from the source, through the top of your head. Visualize your breast filling with that light. Visualize your arm, your armpit, all the way down to your fingers on each side. Feel your left breast full of light. Any place the radiation therapy needs to get to will show up. When you visualize your body filling with the light, any cells that contain cancer will subtly block the light. The "eye" of the radiation sees that gap, the lesser light, and is naturally drawn to fill that part with the next level of radiation, which is the therapeutic radiation.

I did just what Chung Fu asked of me, right there, in the moment: "I'm calling to the solar beings, the solar lords, the solar Goddess," I said. "I'm calling Her to fill my body with the light of the sun. With the light of Source from which radiation, all electricity, all light, emanates. I'm taking the position of the light, of the divine being of light. In my human body, I'm bringing that light in, filling every cell up with it. I'm seeing my body as golden, infused with this light. I'm allowing my body to reveal any place or presence that is unhealthy, or cancerous. I'm allowing any cell where there is even a suggestion of sickness to be seen. By my own radiance, these places will be seen as paler, darker, deeper, and more vacuous, so the light is drawn in, as with a vacuum. 'Nature abhors a vacuum,' so anywhere the light is a little dimmer, that is where the radiation will be magnetized."

I felt soothed by the notion of radiation magnetizing to exactly where it was needed, while the powerful light moving through me from the source of the sun protected the rest of my body.

Chung Fu also suggested that I work with particular crystals for additional power and support during this treatment period. I am a lover of the crystal, rock, and mineral kingdom and greatly benefit from the energies of stones. When I'm preparing for travel, I scan my crystals and ask inside, *Who wants to come with me?* I will inevitably feel drawn to particular stones as soon as I ask this question; one or two will alight with a glow, or my eye will land on a select few. From my travel experience, I've learned that something always happens to confirm why I chose the stones that I did.

About a year ago, my friend Lui, who owns a wonderful crystal shop in Glastonbury, told me he felt shungite and Libyan gold tektite were the most important stones for me to be working with. I carried both with me in my purse. In the rush to evacuate from the fire, I had not had time to bring any of my crystals. I felt unprepared to begin radiation without them until, synchronistically, Chung Fu said the most important stones for me to work with during radiation were in fact the ones I had with me: shungite and Libyan gold. He described shungite as an extraterrestrial crystal that had the power to absorb excess radiation; it was important for me to hold the shungite crystal in my hand during treatments. Libyan gold would fill me up with golden light and bring nourishment to my being, aligning me with solar power. He spoke about the crystalline beings who work through both stones. A crystalline being is a guide or spirit keeper who works through the conduit of a particular stone. Amonshungine is the being who works through the stone shungite to bring protection and draw out negative or harmful energies.

Chung Fu continued to offer additional insight and I flowed with it, knowing he always had my back, had always brought me spiritual offerings from across the realms that helped me move forward, and more importantly, fueled me with calmness, trust and inner strength.

> ***Chung Fu:*** *Amonshungine is a male being, very yang, and very powerful. We say male in the sense that it's very yang power, but actually, it's not really male only. The thing to understand is that the shungite is a strong ally of the human being of this time. This extraterrestrial energy that's being discovered and revealed on your Earth is a powerful evolutionary energy. Your dis-ease is very much the dis-ease of your time. This crystal, that wasn't found that long ago, is a tool that can be used to help draw out poisons in the cancer experience.*
>
> *Once the radiation has done its job, where does it go? Unfortunately, it starts wandering about the body. You're going to use the properties of the shungite to absorb all excess and unnecessary radiation. After each treatment, at the end of the day, you're going to put the shungite in running water, under the tap, for ten or fifteen minutes. Just let the water run over the stone. This will clear all the remaining radiation and any vibration in you that is clinging to the radiation.*
>
> *Shungite will not only draw out excessive radiation, but it will also draw out any other imbalanced energies within your body, such as exhaustion from the radiation process, or shock from the fires. It's okay if you keep the stone with you at night. Allow it to absorb whatever it needs to absorb, followed by the practice of cleansing it before reusing it. This process activates the shungite crystals to a very high vibratory level. Once they absorb what they need, they'll be full and will need to discharge quickly. If you had the time, you could simply leave them out in the rain, or even out in the sun to help them release the charge from*

what they've absorbed. But for now, just use the running water to clear them at the end of the day.

Here is another visualization for you to practice. You're a woman made of the sun, with huge solar energy radiating in your being. Think of the name Aaronata, the feminine essence of Libyan gold. All substances begin as light, and quite often, they become liquid and then crystallize and become solid. I want you to think of Libyan gold as a very powerful liquid that emanates from another dimension. Imagine Aaronata as a goddess. She's a crystal being, but I want you to imagine her as having the power of a goddess. You're calling to Aaronata to be your ally, to fill the whole of your being with her transparent presence of sparkling, flowing gold. Imagine her essence coming through your arteries and veins, flowing into you from the earth, up through the hara, or womb center. The spirit being of Libyan gold, Aaronata, is coming from around you and through your crown.

I resonated with the idea of an ancient, golden goddess infusing me with liquid light. As Chung Fu spoke, I felt warm light flowing through my body, filling my left side—my implant, all of the skin, tissues, and areas that would be receiving radiation. The Libyan gold was a tool to support my body to fill up with light, while the shungite would help draw out excess radiation, heat, and negative energies.

Every day as I go in for treatment, I hold one of these crystals in each hand and think, *As I squeeze the shungite in my right hand, I command Amonshungine to form a shungite shield behind my chest wall in front of my heart and lungs.*

I visualize an impenetrable black wall covering my esophagus and thyroid gland, wrapping around my heart and lungs, and creating a barrier between my two breasts. Through my left hand, I feel a river of sparkling golden light flowing through me. I see my left breast as a castle guarded by thick, black stone walls, with a golden mote surrounding it. The only energies allowed to enter the castle are the ones most supportive and healing to the queen. I am the queen.

. . .

During this time, Chung Fu recommended I take a homeopathic remedy called radiotherapy mix 30c once a day throughout the five weeks of treatment to mitigate some of the side effects. I ordered it from a pharmacy in London, but it hadn't arrived by the first week of treatment, and I experienced fierce headaches and nausea following the radiation. As soon as I began taking the homeopathic remedy, however, the side effects subsided and didn't return. Radiation causes inflammation, and as the weeks went by, my skin became a scalding red color and was hot to the touch. I regularly visited the hyperbaric oxygen chamber; that was a massive support on many levels. From the time I entered the chamber to ninety minutes after my session ended, my flaming red skin faded in color. I could literally feel the inflammation lessening in my body. The doctors consistently commented on how well my skin was doing, which I couldn't believe because to me it still looked horribly burned.

On the final day of treatment, I lie topless with my arms positioned stiffly above my head and my feet bound together, alive in the crucible of fire. My chest, collarbone, entire left breast, and armpit are scorched. My skin is once again blood red, raw; stabbing pains flutter across the burned places, like a symphony of hot needles. I feel as if I could go up in flames, I am so hot. A memory floods into my consciousness, and I am consumed by a scene in which I'm in a similar position:

My body is tied to a wooden stake, and I am naked. The stake is upright, and I am on display for all the townspeople to see, in the center of the town square. No one is helping me; no one will even look into my eyes. A fire is lit at my feet and I am writhing in terror and rage. I scream; I cry out for help as the smoke begins to rise. I am struggling and fighting even though I know I can't change the situation when, without warning, in the midst of my blinding fear and useless cries for help, something shifts inside me. A wave of peace flows over me like a high vibration of love, and I say aloud to myself, "I surrender." I let go completely, allowing the flames to engulf me. My mind is empty, and I feel myself floating on a cloud of deep peace.

Beeping noises pull me out of this blissful state, and temporarily confused, I remember they're coming from the radiation machine. But now, I can feel the purifying quality of the fire; the fire that burned me on the stake is the same fire burning me now. The woman from my past is reaching out to me, bridging our healing across time. She needs me to remember her so the old wounds incurred by fire may be released along with any trace of dis-ease. We were both alone on the stake and here we are now, alone, bound in the very same way. My body surrenders completely, simultaneously in my memory and in the present, and I feel a cleansing energy washing through me. The machine goes quiet, and I hear a voice within clearly speak, "All karma related to breast cancer is now absolved through the purification of fire. The absolution is complete. It is done."

The next time I spoke with Chung Fu, I shared my cleansing-by-fire encounter and found his response sensitive and thoroughly resonant, as usual.

Chung Fu: Your body is releasing very deep wounds at the moment. The radiation, the burning, is triggering betrayals from other lives to rise to the surface. You've lived many priestess lives, and in your present life, this unrecognized child, who is a seer child, came in with a traumatic childhood. In the priestess life you glimpsed, which was also very traumatic, you surrendered, and that made the burning go quicker, but you actually didn't die of the burning; you died of the fumes. Fire rapidly consumes oxygen and you couldn't breathe. That's the moment of letting go that you remember.

I knew he was right. That was exactly what it felt like to me—a fast, yet intense, struggle, and then I couldn't move. In my mind's eye, I see this woman who burned at the stake and honor her, thanking her for showing herself to me. She is free now, her pain no longer bound within my body.

INANNA'S ASCENT

Gate 2: Retrieves Her Lapis Necklace: I Am Light

Inanna ascends through the second gate of the underworld, retrieving her lapis necklace. As she places the familiar jewels upon her skin, she is aware that although they helped to empower her connection with her third eye, her inner vision, or spiritual sight, was inside her all along. Buying into the idea that she needed this necklace to connect with her innate gifts actually created the illusion that her gifts were being held at a distance, away from her. In the dark of the underworld, she learned to access her own eternal light of truth. She touches the lapis and smiles, feeling the energy pulsing on her brow like a dancing candle flame.

I had believed that my beloved Blue was my conduit to my truest self, to the magical seer child within me. Blue had opened a gateway to help me remember what was there all along but had been hidden and suppressed. My journey into the underworld led me to my inner nature, reawakening the magical young girl inside, whose vision is crystal clear. If I could connect to my wild inner nature and the magical essence of my being in the most sterile, cold medical environment imaginable, strapped down under a machine on a metal slab with no one else in the room, then I could do it anywhere. I no longer needed the physical representation of something outside me to grant access or permission to my inner vision.

As I walk through the second gate of the underworld, I feel illuminated, filled with the golden light of the sun.

· · ·

While spiritually I felt sparkling and full of light, physically, mentally, and emotionally I was exhausted. My body was still in shock from the cumulative treatments, and I still hurt from the burns. I began to regularly recite a Hawaiian prayer called the Hopono'pono, placing my hands over my left breast and saying aloud, "I love you. I'm sorry, please forgive me. Thank you." I continued to visualize golden light streaming in and filling my body with love. Chung Fu's message flooded my mind:

> *One of the great teachings of cancer is that you don't get to survive unless you love yourself. This is a test you're passing through. Your entire healing process is to practice self-love. For you, cancer has been a big hit on the mother area. The left breast is about supreme Divine Mother. Your healing began with your inner child, telling her she's safe—you did it, together. Feel her included in all, enabling her to have faith in her own inner mother.*

JOURNAL ENTRY

Last night, with my skin so very badly burned and intense stabbing pain, I felt raw, both in my body and in my spirit. Completely vulnerable and uncomfortable, I had a desire to crawl into Ryan's lap. I wanted to be small. My body wanted to be small. I wanted to curl up on top of him and have all of me fit onto him. I had a visceral memory of being a child, able to curl up on my dad's lap and fit, like a cat. I wanted this so badly. I wanted to be held by my dad as a little kid.

I'm realizing how scared my "little girl" is going through this and how much I need to comfort her. I asked inside, What does she need? She wants Penny (her golden retriever) and a chocolate ice cream cone. I pictured all three of us outside Cravings in Charlevoix, Michigan (a childhood summertime ice cream shop)—me with my chocolate ice cream, Penny, and my dad. This was supremely comforting.

Only two more treatments left.

JOURNAL PROMPT

How would your view of the world change if you saw it through the wonder-filled eyes of a child? What if magic is indeed all around us?

MEDITATION

Sit comfortably with your spine straight, or lie down, where you will not be disturbed. Close your eyes, and begin taking in deep diaphragmatic breaths, in through the nose, filling and expanding the belly, and out through the mouth with an audible exhale...ahhh. Repeat three times.

Visualize yourself standing on a beautiful forest path. Looking out into the distance, you see the silhouette of two figures walking toward you, one adult and one child. As they get closer, you recognize Inanna, and to your delight, you see that she is walking hand in hand with your inner child. This child is brimming with joy, eyes alight, with a big smile. Running toward you, your inner child embraces you with deep love. Allow yourself to receive the child's loving presence, innocence, and purity. You notice your child has a gift for you, and they offer it to you with excitement. Your child has retrieved something significant from deep within your memory, so that you may recall what you loved dearly as a child. This may be a game, a toy, a childhood playmate, a beloved pet, a tree, an imaginary friend, a song, a story you loved, or anything that comes into your awareness. As you open this gift, you are filled with the remembrance of a magical world, one where anything is possible. This gift opens a gateway to your magical inner world, where you may connect with the essence of your inner child at any time. This inner world of imagination is where you may access your inner vision and connect with your deepest and most expansive dreams for your life. Make an agreement with your inner child that you will honor them by tending to this sacred place within you.

Give thanks to Inanna and your precious child, holding your child in reverence and gratitude, giving them a nice cuddle. Exchange any words you would like to speak, perhaps letting them know you love them and that you will always be here for them.

When you are ready, take in a few deep belly breaths and place your hands on your body, inviting yourself to anchor back in the present moment.

Open your eyes and journal any insights that came forward.

Blessed be.

Chapter Fourteen

WHOLENESS

FIRST GATE: CROWN OF GLORY

"No problem can be solved from the same level of
consciousness that created it."

~ Albert Einstein

I have always resonated with Einstein's quote about not being able
to solve a problem from the level it was created. I believe this to be
true about many things in life, especially healing. When faced with
a serious or life-threatening illness, one must open to explore new
pathways toward healing and self-awareness, approaching the situation from a fresh perspective. The most immediate shift comes when
we are able to ask ourselves, "Why is this happening *for* me?" instead
of, "Why is this happening *to* me?" I was determined to utilize my
illness as an opportunity for learning more about myself. I saw cancer as a vehicle through which my soul was seeking wholeness. I was
being asked to recalibrate to a higher level of awareness to remember
all that I am, *wholly*.

I finished one year of treatment on the eve of the winter solstice,
after having begun light infusions the previous January 2. Between

January and April, I received six rounds of light infusions, during which I received four different medicines. Two of these were chemo drugs, while the other two were considered therapeutic medicines and didn't have the violent side effects of chemo. I continued receiving these two medications via IV infusion every three weeks for the duration of the year. One of these medications is called Herceptin, a drug that changed the prognosis for women diagnosed as HER2 positive, as I was, from a formidable diagnosis to a favorable one because the drug is so effective. Many times, while receiving this medicine, I wept in gratitude for the courageous women who came before me and went through the clinical trials to make this drug available to me. I also wept for the women who, twenty years ago, were not as fortunate.

As emotional as I was going through treatment, as the light returned after the darkest night of the year, I also began to see how numb I had become. Enduring regular treatments required rigorous strength and a slight disconnection from my body. I had been repeatedly envisioning myself as a warrior goddess with a sword and shield. Each time the nurse prepared my IV, I would close my eyes and hear the clanking of my sword against the shield and see my face painted in blood. I felt other warrior sisters and brothers around me, my tribe, grunting and growling, emanating primal power. Without the presence of the treatments as a reason to hold onto my strength, I began to notice that I was emotionally covered in heavy, metal armor. I was living in a fortress built to protect me from the constant battle of not only the invasive procedures but the intensely stressful conversations with doctors speaking in statistics about the chances of my survival. Disarming the armor was as much of an emotional roller coaster as erecting it had been. My oncologist had prepared me by saying that most people warrior through chemo, surgery, and radiation, counting the days until they can get their life back, only to realize they are no longer the same person, and that life will never be the same. As consciously as I tried to move through that year of treatment, a heavy grief still met me on the other side, full of deep mourning for the woman I had been before.

I was shell-shocked. I didn't know how to relate to anyone. I had traveled through time and space, existing completely in other worlds and dimensions, and was returning completely disoriented, like a time traveler who doesn't know what year it is. The medical reality was as much its own world as my underworld cave. For self-preservation, I had been navigating only the medically specific realms, with very little contact with the outside world. When I finished treatment, it struck me to hear people say, "Oh you're done! Great! So glad you're better now." I knew this was well-intentioned, but it felt minimizing of something immeasurably complex. Perhaps physically I was "done" with the most grueling challenges, but psychologically I did not feel "better." I was experiencing high levels of anxiety, panic attacks, and feelings of dread, imagining the next terrible thing that might happen. I went to a compassionate hypnotherapist who let me know I was dealing with textbook posttraumatic stress. I was greatly relieved to receive the tools he offered me, and my number one priority became protecting my body from stress, no matter what. This looked like doing less, taking things off my plate, and allowing myself plenty of time to accomplish the things I chose. If something was beginning to cause stress, I needed to stop, cancel, or reschedule. I learned to take cues from my nervous system and be very gentle and forgiving with myself. Meditation, daily exercise, and being out in nature were more important than ever for me.

I also worked regularly with an incredibly skilled body worker who supported me in releasing trauma. I lay on her table as layers of wounds, shock, and suffering unleashed, uncoiling from the places where it had clung to my fascia and tissues, storing pockets of old energy and emotion. Sometimes it came out as moans, yells, or screams. Sometimes laughter or tears. Sometimes my body trembled.

After countless hours researching various detox methods, diets, and preventive protocols, I was guided to yet another wonderful doctor, Dr. Leigh Erin Connealy. She continued to support me in healing my body from the effects of chemo, surgery, and radiation. Dr. Connealy's focus was on healing the underlying imbalances that were present in my body before the illness, as well as active cancer prevention. She taught me that the definition of remission or cure is zero circulating tumor cells, which is not commonly tested for in medical practice. She *does* test for this and creates a highly individualized protocol to eradicate any of those circulating cells. I felt aligned with and empowered by her comprehensive, integrative approach. Coffee enemas, mistletoe injections, high-dose vitamin C IVs, ozone treatments, lymphatic drainage, infrared sauna, cold plunges, and a plethora of daily supplements became part of my regular routine. After years of internalized dogma around diet, I began to deeply listen to what my body was asking for, beyond the programmed ideas of what was okay for me and what was not, according to an outside source. I love eating intuitively and nourishing my body with fresh, organic, plant-focused, seasonal whole foods.

As I rise and discover who I am on the other side of this journey, my most constant companion is gratitude. Gratitude for the precious gift of life. For every sunrise and sunset, for the majestic presence of the moon, for the earth beneath my feet, for every breath. For sacred moments shared, for the profound resilience and healing power of my body, for cuddles with my purring kitties, for deep belly laughs, for tears shed when something touches my heart, for the nurturing touch of a loved one. For the privilege of feeling angry, sad, joyful, excited, or ecstatic. For the gift of being an emotional being, for the ability to ride the tides of my life and feel deeply. When I'm tired, I rest. When I don't feel like doing something, I sit it out. When I feel my soul calling me to try something new, I dive in. I give myself permission to let the wisdom of my body lead.

INANNA'S ASCENT

Gate 1: Retrieves Her Crown: Wholeness

Inanna prepares to walk across the threshold that separates the world below from the one above. As she approaches the first gate of the underworld, she turns to face me. We stare into each other's eyes, soulfully communicating lifetimes of understanding between us. She lovingly places her hand on my heart, and touching my reconstructed breast, reminds me that *no one leaves the underworld unmarked*. I nod knowingly and watch as she retrieves her crown, the beautiful jeweled headpiece that had represented so much to her before. She now knows that her queendom flows through her. She *is* the crown. She is one with the sacred source of life; she is the light of the stars; she *is* Goddess. Following in her footsteps, brimming with gratitude for having her as my guide, I understand that for me, the real crown is my transformation. Losing my hair catapulted me into an amazing journey, one in which I was given the opportunity to fully embody my strength as a woman. I have walked through fire, turning lead into gold at every turn and emerging fully as my priestess self. I have traveled through the mists and back, bridging time and space, retrieving the magical essence that is my birthright. As I ascend through the first gate, which aligns with the spiritual energy center at the top of my head, I know my prayers have been answered. The crown chakra is where our prayers, as well as the prayers others send to us, are held. Physical beauty may be fleeting, but the beauty of the soul is eternal.

In shedding old perceptions of beauty and ways of defining myself as a woman, I have released limiting belief systems that falsely told me how to behave to feel safe or receive approval. I have let go of lifetimes of fear, grief, and pain. Out of the murky waters of my unconscious, I have reclaimed parts of myself that had been disowned. I have unearthed power I had lost and integrated its strength into my conscious awareness. I have expanded into the understanding that *I am one with all that is.* The humanness of my journey has shown me my innate divinity. I am simultaneously human and divine. I am the living embodiment of Goddess, the Lady of the Lake.

I remember going to see Jim George for the first time, a few weeks after being diagnosed. At that time, I communicated that my intention was to liberate myself into wholeness. In that first session, he asked me if I knew the definition of the word *heal*. He shared that it means "to make whole," stemming from the root, *haelan,* which he defined as "the condition or state of being whole, or hal." Hal is the root of the word *holy.*

My healing came from recognizing myself as holy.

I am healed

I am whole

I am holy

Blessed be

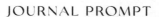

JOURNAL PROMPT

What prayers in your life have been answered? How would it feel to know yourself as holy?

MEDITATION

Sit comfortably with your spine straight, or lie down, where you will not be disturbed. Close your eyes, and begin taking in deep diaphragmatic breaths, in through the nose, filling and expanding the belly, and out through the mouth with an audible exhale...ahhh. Repeat three times.

Visualize the goddess Inanna standing before you, in her regal glory, adorned in her crown. This is the first time you've seen her wearing all her regalia, and even though she is a beautiful sight, your attention is drawn most powerfully to her presence. She is embodied, filled with truth, wisdom, and self-love. As she stands before you, she offers you a symbol, a representation of your healing and wholeness. See this symbol floating in the air, vibrating between your hearts as you face one another. Take in a deep breath and feel your body and energy field receiving the frequency of this symbol, inviting the healing power to go wherever it is needed.

When you are ready, Inanna cups her hands around your sacred symbol and begins directing it upward toward your crown. Lifting it higher and higher, she places your symbol above your head, into the energy center of your crown. This is a symbol of your power, sovereignty, divinity, and wholeness. This symbol opens a channel through which you will always be connected to your highest Self and truth, a reminder that you are always held and protected by the Divine, and that spiritual support and guidance are always available to you. Breathe and become aware of any shifts that may be taking place as your energy field recalibrates to receive the power of this symbol.

When you are ready, express your gratitude to Inanna for her guidance and support along this journey. Begin to feel your feet, wiggling your toes and rubbing your hands together to bring yourself back into your body. Placing your hands on your belly, take in a few deep grounding breaths. Slowly open your eyes and draw your healing symbol. Journal any insights that came forward.

Blessed be.

CLOSING

By the earth that is Her body
By the air that is Her breath
By the fire of Her bright spirit
And the waters of Her living womb
The circle is open but unbroken
May the peace of the Goddess be forever in your heart
Merry meet, and merry part, and merry meet again.

~ Prayer spoken at the closing of goddess ceremonies around the world

Dear sister, brother, friend. If you are currently facing a serious or life-threatening diagnosis, know that within your outer circumstances there is an inner opportunity to know yourself as holy. You are not alone. You walk with all the beings you have been and all that you shall be. You are being called to remember your divinity, to embrace the magic within you. You are being asked to let go of all that has kept those memories from you, so that you may dismantle the patriarchy within you and see through the falsehoods that have indoctrinated our culture for lifetimes.

Rage sister, rage. Scream, cry, and discharge the energies of suppression, betrayal, and all that has hurt you and held you captive from your truth.

Feminine dis-ease is a calling to personally and collectively heal the sacred feminine. On a soul level, you have a mission to heal on a larger scale, and through your journey, you will be able to release collective and ancestral pain. *You have the strength for this.* You have all the inner resources you need to navigate the path that lies ahead. If the purpose of life is to grow and evolve spiritually, as I believe it is, you are being presented with your greatest material toward liberation.

Find a spiritual healer, spiritual counselor, shamanic practitioner, or soul-centered therapist who can help light the way for you as you courageously face and walk through these dark and fiery places. To locate this person, send out a call from your heart to your higher Self, your ancient and future selves, and all beings who support you, asking them to please bring the people into your life who are meant to be part of your healing team. Trust you will be guided to the right people, and they will also be led to you. May you know deep in your bones who is meant to support you. Remember, this is not about accommodating others—every choice is *for* you and your healing, *not against* anyone else. May you cry, releasing lifetimes of tears, allowing them to flow through you like cleansing rain.

May you forgive any judgments you have held against yourself.

Create a ceremony to help you cut ties with those who have hurt you, while surrounding your soul and theirs with love and forgiveness. Write down past hurts and bury them in the earth or burn them in a fire. No anger or resentment is worth holding onto when you see how it affects your health.

Make choices in service to life. Affirm life and vitality in your being. Speak your truths from your heart and tell people, places, trees, and animals you love what they mean to you.

Connect with nature as much as possible. Swim in a lake, spring, or ocean, and get your bare feet into the dirt. Sit with your back against a tree, feeling your own roots descending deep into the soil, grounding and nourishing you, releasing and transmuting any toxicity. Spend time in the moonlight and under the stars, opening to receive the mysteries that are held in the dark places. Soak up the sunshine, allowing the light to illuminate your being. You have the power to choose the way you relate to every experience you encounter in your life. Everything can be sacred. Everything can be made beautiful.

Feel my hands reaching out through these pages to hold yours, now, at this very moment. I stand before you in flowing sapphire-colored priestess robes, a crescent moon painted upon my brow. Beside me to my left there is a chalice, and to my right, a sword. As I dip my fingers in the silver chalice, which is engraved with a triple spiral, I anoint your brow with holy water.

May your inner vision be open.

May you be guided gracefully to the perfect people who are meant to support your healing journey.

May you trust yourself every step of the way, making each decision from deep within.

May the inner pathways open for you to remember who you truly are as a divine being.

I reach to my right and take hold of the base of the sword that is adorned with aquamarine jewels. As I remove the sheath that is carved with ancient symbols, the shining blade is revealed. I hold the sword in front of your body, the base at your root chakra, between your legs, with the tip of the sword at your crown.

May you be in alignment with your soul's highest truth.

May you awaken the sovereign being within, facing this journey with courage and conviction.

May you experience clarity and discernment as you face the unknown.

May you be surrounded with divine protection now and always.

As you walk the path of your own journey, I affirm these truths for you:

You are healed.

You are whole.

You are holy.

You are a unique emanation of the Divine,

a living embodiment of Goddess.

Blessed be.

GRATITUDE

So many beautiful beings supported me in the creation of this book.

I would first like to thank my wonderful writing coach, Parthenia M. Hicks, who patiently guided me in expressing and shaping the language of my inner world. Huge thanks to Darnah and my awesome team at Scribe Publishing.

I give thanks to my amazing family; I love you all so dearly. I especially acknowledge Nana, Mimi, Amy, Sheila, Wells, Remy, and my extraordinary parents, Kate and Stephen. To my Mom and Dad, I am so grateful I chose you both. Thank you for your unconditional love and support and for honoring the powerful sacred contracts our souls signed up for. To Michael, thank you for your loving encouragement and for always seeing me in my radiant health and vitality.

I offer my deepest, most heartfelt gratitude for my beautiful sisters who were in my prayer circle, and who continue to hold me so strongly and tenderly through this sacred journey of life: April Rucker, Val Dillman, Keri Lassalle, Bonne Chance, Ashley Smith, Maura Moynihan Amoroso, Angela Escamillas, Sunder Ashni, Gigi Chiarello, Baelyn Elspeth, Jenny Emblom Castro, Harmony Marya, and Caroline Corcoran. I give thanks to Kaycee Flinn, for the blessing of many years of loving sisterhood, and to Jessica Karr, for being such a magical friend. I give thanks to Melissa Barron; you are an inspiration and way shower. I give thanks to Ryan Russell for your loving care and support, for being the man of integrity that you are, and for the wonderful illustration in the beginning of this book.

Big hugs to the sisters of Her Sacred Waters 2019, Mara Luasa Elaine, Dreesie, Molly Bloom, Hermas, Regan, Lindsey Mac, Sri Mati, Jade Rose, Libby, Hana, Camilla, Marcelle, Graell, Leonora, WuDe and Joyce and the Global Tea Hut family, and the wonderful community of women who attend my ceremonies in person and online.

Many healers and guides played significant roles in my journey, including my beloved horse, Blue; my magical healing cats and soul companions, Maddie and Clark; spiritual counselor Alisha Das; oracle and trance medium Sally Pullinger and the Chung Fu family, Sophie and Jerome; priestess teachers, sisters, friends, and mentors Luna Silver and Kathy Jones; friend and guide Jim George; oncologist Dr. Laurence Piro and his caring nurses and staff; breast surgeon Dr. Kristi Funk; reconstructive surgeon Dr. Tiffany Grunwald; doctor of Chinese medicine Dr. Dao; Dr. Leigh Erin Connealy at Cancer Center for Healing; and, of course, my unseen guides and helpers, the unconditional love of Goddess, and the Lady of the Lake.

I honor and give thanks to my beautiful priestess family and community in Avalon, and acknowledge Heloise, Annabel, John Wadsworth, Sophie Docker, Sue, Savannah, Lui, Tor, Daisy, and all my beloved spiral sisters and dear spiral brother. I give thanks to the land of Avalon, the Lady of Avalon, as well as the spirit of Topanga Canyon and all her land, trees, and creatures.

Extra special thanks to Alisha, April, Keri, and Dawn, for witnessing my writing as it was unfolding and for your unconditional support and encouragement of this book. Extra loving thanks to Bonne and Ash for being the most amazing cheerleaders.

I acknowledge all the teachers and friends who have inspired me along my path with Goddess, including Kyle King, Suzanne Sterling, Gerri Ravyn Stanfield, Starhawk and the Reclaiming Community, Saul David Raye, Laura Amazzone, Sri Mata Amritanandamayi Devi (Amma), Colette Crawford, Ashley Turner, Mara Freeman, and Tami Lynn Kent. Last but not least, I give thanks to Colin for seeing me and giving me the book *The Mists of Avalon* all those years ago. Blessed be.

ABOUT THE
AUTHOR

Annah Taylor Phinny is a spiritual healer and formally trained Priestess of Avalon, an ancient Goddess tradition based in Glastonbury, England. During her teens, her intuitive nature led to nightly readings for her classmates, which in turn led to accusations of witchcraft, expulsion, and medication that suppressed her gifts for many years.

Today, Annah Taylor has completed a master's program in spiritual psychology with an emphasis in consciousness, health, and healing and lives in service to the divine feminine in all beings. Supporting others in connecting with their wild and ancient selves through ceremony, retreats, and pilgrimage is the work she cherishes most. During her transformational journey, Taylor experienced a rebirth, emerging with the name Annah. She is the founder of Avalon Calling, offering pilgrimages to the sacred sites of the British Isles as well as personal and group priestess sessions. To connect with Annah, visit AvalonCalling.co.

RESOURCES

PHYSICAL, MENTAL, EMOTIONAL, AND SPIRITUAL SUPPORT

Dear friend,

I know that looking through lists of resources can be overwhelming, especially when creating your own supportive healthcare plan. I've organized this list into four segments: physical, mental, emotional, and spiritual. To start, I recommend choosing one or two resources from each section. This way, you are working holistically. Before you choose, take a deep breath and ask yourself, What is the best next step for me? Scan the list to see what stands out to you and trust your intuition.

Many blessings on your healing path.

Annah Taylor Phinny

PHYSICAL-LEVEL SUPPORT

Acupuncture

Tao of Wellness Clinics in Los Angeles

~ https://www.taoofwellness.com

Body, Mind, Spirit Cleansing and Detox Program

Hippocrates Health Institute in Palm Beach, Florida

~ https://hippocratesinst.org

Optimum Health Institute in San Diego, CA, and Austin, TX

~ http://www.optimumhealth.org/

Books

Connealy, Dr. Leigh Erin. *The Cancer Revolution: A Groundbreaking Program to Reverse and Prevent Cancer*. New York, NY: Hachette Books, 2017.

Fayed, Camilla. *Farmacy Kitchen Cookbook: Plant-Based Recipes for a Conscious Way of Life*. Aster, 2018.

Funk, Dr. Kristi. *Breasts: The Owner's Manual: Every Woman's Guide to Reducing Cancer Risk, Making Treatments Choices, and Optimizing Outcomes*. Harlequin Mills & Boon, Limited, 2018.

Gainsley, Lisa Levitt. *The Book of Lymph; Self-Care Lymphatic Massage to Enhance Immunity, Health, and Beauty*. Harper Wave, 2021.

Piatt, Julie. *The Plant Power Way: Whole Food Plant-Based Recipes & Guidance for the Whole Family: A Cookbook*. Avery, 2015.

Wynters, Sharyn, ND, and Burton Goldberg, LHD. *The Pure Cure: A Complete Guide to Freeing Your Life from Dangerous Toxins*. Berkeley, CA: Soft Skull Press, 2012.

Cancer Care and Prevention—Highly Individualized and Progressive

~ https://www.cancercenterforhealing.com

Documentary Films

~ https://www.earthingmovie.com

~ https://thecwordmovie.vhx.tv

Holistic Approaches to Cleansing and Diet

Books and Podcast by Anthony William

~ https://www.medicalmedium.com

Breast Cancer Conqueror Podcast with Dr. V

~ https://breastcancerconqueror.com

Coffee Enemas: Be sure to use organic coffee specifically for enemas (can order from this link) and speak to your physician first. Not to be done during chemo or radiation.

~ https://www.purelifeenema.com/about-coffee-enemas/

Hormonal Support

Lots of informative articles by Dr. Jolene Brighten

~ https://drbrighten.com

Homeopathy

~ https://www.ainsworths.com

~ https://www.smhomeopathic.com/store/

Infrared Amethyst BioMat

~ https://www.biomat.com

Lymphatic Health

Follow Lisa Levitt Gainsley on Instagram, where she shares informative videos about lymphatic self-massage.

~ https://www.thelymphaticmessage.com

Mushrooms for Immunity

~ https://hostdefense.com

Nipple Tattooing

~ https://www.huffpost.com/entry/
nipple-tattoos-breast-cancer_n_5bcf6350e4b0d38b587d07e9

Pilates Online

~ https://www.pilatesbysorel.com

Practical Support While Going through Cancer Treatment

~ https://cancer.livebetterwith.
com/#shopify-section-1551877243156

Quantum Resonance System (QRS), pulsed electromagnetic field product (PEMF)

~ https://www.qrs.com

Trauma Release Technique

~ https://traumaprevention.com/

Yoga Online

~ https://www.gaia.com

~ https://www.glo.com

Look for These Healing Therapies in Your Area

~ Acupuncture

~ Bodywork—You'll know you've found a skilled bodyworker who's in alignment with your healing if you feel a shift in your mind/body/spirit after the session.

~ Cold plunge

~ Headscarves—If you're looking for headscarves, ask friends to let you borrow ones they love, or perhaps make a trip to a local thrift store to find something fun.

~ Hyperbaric oxygen chamber

~ Infrared sauna

MENTAL-LEVEL SUPPORT

Books

Dispenza, Dr. Joe. *Becoming Supernatural: How Common People Are Doing the Uncommon*. Carlsbad, CA: Hay House, Inc, 2017.

~ See also: Joe Dispenza online courses, downloadable meditations, and videos: https://drjoedispenza.com

George, Jim. *Time to Make It Stop: The How of Now*. James Lloyd George III, 2011.

Lipton, Bruce. *The Biology of Belief: Unleashing the Power of Consciousness, Matter & Miracles*. Carlsbad, CA: Hay House, Inc, 2016.

Singer, Micheal. *The Untethered Soul: The Journey beyond Yourself.* New Harbinger Publications, 2007.

BrainTap—Optimizing Brain Health

~ https://braintap.com

Byron Katie

Free downloads, videos, books, and an app

~ https://thework.com

Cancer Personality

~ http://www.alternative-cancer-care.com/the-cancer -personality.html

Documentary Film

~ https://www.healdocumentary.com

Global Tea Hut

Learn the art of tea meditation.

~ https://globalteahut.org

Meditation App

~ https://www.calm.com

~ https://insighttimer.com

Podcast Episode with Stillness Meditation Master Jim George

~ https://www.youtube.com/watch?v=hY4oUCq1b4I

10-minute guided meditation with Jim George

~ https://www.youtube.com/watch?v=iyWrBrFEtd4

Look for These Healing Therapies in Your Area

~ Hypnotherapy

~ Meditation classes

~ Psilocybin therapy

~ Tea ceremony

EMOTIONAL-LEVEL SUPPORT

Books

Estes, Clarissa Pinkola, PhD. *Women Who Run with the Wolves: Myths and Stories of the Wild Woman Archetype*. Ballantine Books, 1996.

Hay, Louise. *You Can Heal Your Life*. Carlsbad, CA: Hay House, Inc, 1984.

Hulnick, H. Ronald, PhD, and Mary R. Hulnick, PhD. *Loyalty to Your Soul: The Heart of Spiritual Psychology*. Carlsbad, CA: Hay House, Inc., 2011.

———. *Remembering the Light Within: A Course in Soul-Centered Living*. Carlsbad, CA: Hay House, Inc., 2017.

Nelson, Dr. Bradley. *The Emotion Code: How to Release Your Trapped Emotions for Abundant Health, Love, and Happiness*. St. Martin's Essentials, 2019.

Paul, Margaret. *The Inner Bonding Workbook: Six Steps to Healing Yourself and Connecting with Your Divine Guidance*. Oakland: Reveal Press, 2019.

LADY OF THE LAKE, RISE

Thomashauer, Regina. *Pussy: A Reclamation*. Carlsbad, CA: Hay House, Inc., 2016.

Breathwork

~ https://revelationbreathwork.com

~ https://www.somabreath.com

Deep Inner Work on All Levels of Consciousness with Annah Taylor

My online course, The Lady's Mirror

~ https://www.avaloncalling.co/ladys-mirror

Flower Essences

~ http://www.bachflower.com

~ https://chalicewell.org.uk/product-category/
  chalice-well-essences/

Free-Form Writing

~ https://www.msia.org/experience/free-form-writing

Gestalt Therapy

~ https://www.psychologytoday.com/us/therapy-types/
  gestalt-therapy

Loving and Healing Yourself

~ https://www.innerbonding.com

Programs in Spiritual Psychology

~ http://www.universityofsantamonica.edu

Shadow Work

~ https://www.robertmasters.com

Somatic Experiencing

~ https://traumahealing.org/resources/

~ https://youtu.be/nmJDkzDMllc

The Class—Online Exercise Focused on Emotional and Somatic Release

~ https://www.theclass.com

Look for These Healing Therapies in Your Area

~ Breathwork

~ Ecstatic Dance

~ Rage Room

SPIRITUAL-LEVEL SUPPORT

Astrology

Astrology courses online and in the United Kingdom, personal chart readings

~ http://www.kairosastrology.co.uk

Online astrology classes, personal chart readings, weekly horoscopes

~ https://divineharmony.com

Goddess-centered astrology with a Priestess of Avalon

~ https://www.stellarmysteryschool.com

Avalon Calling Community—Ladies of the Lake Membership

Includes monthly live circles with Annah as well as opportunities for one-on-one sessions, retreats, and pilgrimages to Avalon

~ https://avalon-calling.mn.co

Link to invite page; I hope to see you there!

~ https://avalon-calling.mn.co/share/B8Mx3UvogmapDykJ

Books

Ingerman, Sandra. *Soul Retrieval: Mending the Fragmented Self.* New York, NY: Harper One, 2006.

Jones, Kathy. *Priestess of Avalon, Priestess of the Goddess*. Riverside, CA: Ariadne Publications, 2006.

Mercier, David. *A Beautiful Medicine: A Radical Look at the Essence of Health*. Still Bond Press, 2012.

Myss, Caroline. *Anatomy of the Spirit: The Seven Stages of Power and Healing*. New York, NY: Penguin Random House, 1996.

———. *Why People Don't Heal and How They Can*, New York, NY: Random House/Three Rivers Press, 1997.

Queen Afua. *Sacred Woman: A Guide to Healing the Feminine Body, Mind, and Spirit*. United Kingdom: One World, 2001.

Rasha. *Oneness*, 2nd Edition. Santa Fe, NM: Earthstar press, 2006.

Starhawk. *The Spiral Dance: A Rebirth of the Ancient Religion of the Goddess*. New York, NY: Harper Collins, 1979, 1989, 1999.

Wadsworth, John. *Your Zodiac Soul: Working with the Twelve Zodiac Gateways to Create Balance, Happiness, and Wholeness*. New York, NY: Hachette Book Group, 2018.

Wolkstein, Diane & Samuel Noah Kramer. *Inanna: Queen of Heaven and Earth*. New York, NY: Harper & Row 1983.

Documentary Film

The Healing Field: Exploring Energy and Consciousness on Amazon Prime or Gaia

~ https://www.amazon.com/Healing-Field-Exploring-Consciousness-Expanded/dp/B075GVGXJG

Dream Work

~ https://www.dreamingwithval.com

Earth-Based Spirituality and Witchcraft

Reclaiming Collective

~ https://reclaimingcollective.wordpress.com/reclaiming-tradition-witchcraft/

Expanding Consciousness

~ https://energeticsynthesis.com

~ https://veilofreality.com

Goddess Temples

Glastonbury Goddess Temple

~ https://goddesstemple.co.uk

Goddess Temple of Ashland, Oregon

~ https://www.goddesstempleashland.com

Healing Crystals and Sacred Adornments

~ https://www.stoneage.co.uk

Inanna—Venus

Annabel's Rose Moon Membership works with the ancient Venus-Moon Cycle

~ https://annabelduboulay.com

Sacred Sound Healing

~ https://www.heloisepilkington.com

Sacred Sound and Shungite Crystals

~ www.jrokka.com

Shamanic Healing and Mediumship

Live Teleseminars, Online Courses, and Sessions with Chung Fu

~ http://www.deepsoulconnection.com

Remote Shamanic Sessions

~ https://iamaprilrucker.com

Spiritual Counselors

Alisha Das and Michael Hayes
Check out their YouTube channel for free videos.

~ http://awaketolove.com

Learn more about Alisha's offerings here:

~ https://alishadas.com

Spiritual Service Livestream

~ https://agapelive.com

~ https://michaelbeckwith.com

Look for These Healing Therapies in Your Area

~ Crystal Healing

~ Energy Healing

~ Sound Healing/Sound Baths

~ Spiritual Counseling